Orotic Acid

Orotic Acid

Alois Čihák PhD

Institute of Organic Chemistry and Biochemistry, Czechoslovakia Academy of Sciences Prague, Czechoslovakia

and

Werner Reutter MD

Institut für Molekularbiologie und Biochemie der Freien
Universität, Berlin, Germany

SPRINGER SCIENCE+BUSINESS MEDIA, LLC

Published by

MTP Press Limited
Falcon House
Lancaster, England

Copyright © 1980 A.Čihák and W. Reutter

Softcover reprint of the hardcover 1st edition 1980

British Library Cataloguing in Publication Data
    Čihák, Alois Orotic acid.
    1. Orotic acid
    I. Title II. Reutter, Werner
    574.1'924   QP801.0/

ISBN 978-94-009-8045-7   ISBN 978-94-009-8043-3 (eBook)
DOI 10.1007/ 978-94-009-8043-3

Redwood Burn Limited
Trowbridge & Esher

Contents

Preface

This volume reviews a series of different publications dealing with orotic acid. Orotic acid was isolated from cow's milk 75 years ago by Biscaro and Belloni in Italy. Fifty years later again Italian scientists described the growth-promoting activity of orotic acid in vitamin B_{12}-deficient animals. Orotic acid is the precursor of pyrimidine nucleotides which are involved in many biochemical reactions: UTP and CTP, as substrates for RNA polymerase, and UDP sugars, as substrates for carbohydrate containing macromolecules, e.g. glycogen, glycoproteins and glycolipids. The biosynthesis of these pyrimidines is well regulated. Disturbance of the biosynthetic pathway or trapping of individual pyrimidine nucleotides may lead to severe metabolic and structural alterations of cells. Synthesis, biochemical aspects and physiological role are reviewed in nine chapters. In the last two decades increasing interest in orotic acid came from several studies showing protective or therapeutic or beneficial effects of this compound in different kinds of organ injuries: various forms of hepatic insufficiency, myocardial infarction, encephalopathy, memorization processes, mentioned in Chapters 8 and 9.

At the end of this overview a Bibliography in an alphabetical order with 673 references may give further insight in this topic.

A. Čihák
W. Reutter

Orotic Acid:
Synthesis, Biochemical Aspects and Physiological Role

1. New Growth Factor?

Orotic acid was isolated by Biscaro and Belloni [1] in Italy in 1905 from cow's milk where it constitutes the major pyrimidine. While cow's milk and commercial powdered milk [2] have a relatively high content of orotic acid (50–100 mg l^{-1} and 100–130 mg per 100 g protein respectively) human milk contains only trace amounts of orotic acid [3,4]. Its concentration in other foods is not yet known. There are several reports dealing with the amount of orotic acid in milk and milk products (chocolate, food milk powders etc.) [5–12] and several different techniques were developed for the measurement of its concentration [13–16].

Orotic acid

In addition to its importance in the synthesis of nucleic acids and other substances containing pyrimidine, evidence began to accumulate indicating that this 2,6-dioxypyrimidine derivative might be one of the growth factors in animals [17–19]. The physiological role of orotic acid [20–23] was first studied mainly in Italy, Sweden and the United States and later in Germany, Hungary and the Soviet Union (Chapters 8 and 9).

Italian scientists focussed their attention on the growth-promoting action of orotic acid in vitamin B_{12}-deficient rats and chicks [24, 25]. Orotic acid and vitamin B_{12} have similar effects on the metabolism of the C_1-unit, whereby orotic acid increases the concentration of folate derivatives and influences the enzymes involved in the synthesis and utilization of folate intermediates [26,27]. Orotic acid also results in an increase in liver RNA concomitant with the stimulation of nuclear DNA-dependent RNA polymerase activity [28,29]. These findings led to the presumption that orotic acid increases messenger RNA synthesis. There are a number of further reports, mainly from Italy [30–47], dealing with the relationship between orotic acid and vitamin deficiency, distribution and function [48–61].

Orotic acid is used at present as a therapeutic agent in neonatal jaundice, myocardial infarction, and various forms of hepatic insufficiency (Chapter 9). Therapeutic effects of orotic acid have been investigated in a number of conditions, usually with beneficial results, since its administration results in a higher level of pyrimidine precursors of nucleic acids and also the

3

pyrimidine cofactors essential for the conversion of carbohydrates, lipids and some other metabolites. This leads to an increase in the rate and capacity of different metabolic pathways where pyrimidine components are operating, and to the promotion of the growth of the organism [62,63].

In this review several aspects relating to the biochemical and physiological effects of orotic acid will be discussed. Since there are many studies devoted to orotic acid biosynthesis, incorporation, metabolic transformation, physiological and therapeutic roles, only about 500 references, which are believed to cover the main findings, will be presented. Data on the transformation and biological activity of orotic acid (summarized here) can be found elsewhere [20,21,64–69].

References

1. Biscaro, G. and Belloni, E. *Ann. Soc. Chim. Milano*, **11**, 25/5 (1905)
2. Okonkwo, P. O. and Kinsella, J. E. *Am. J. Clin. Nutr.*, **22**, 532 (1969)
3. Kabata, A., Suzuoki, J. and Kide, M. *J. Biochem. (Tokyo)*, **51**, 277 (1962)
4. Hallanger, L. E., Laakso, J. W. and Schultze, M. O. *J. Biol. Chem.*, **202**, 83 (1953)
5. Kieffer, F., Solms, J. and Egli, R. H. *Lebensm. Unters. Forsch.*, **125**, 346 (1964/1965)
6. Kiermeier, F. and Buckl, A. *Lebensm. Unters. Forsch.*, **138**, 284 (1968)
7. Muenchberg, F., Tsompanidou, G. and Leskova, R. *Milchwissenschaft.*, **26**, 210 (1971)
8. Motz, R. J. *Analyst*, **97**, 866 (1972)
9. Archer, A. W. *Analyst*, **98**, 755 (1973)
10. Garcia, O. R., Carballido, A. and Torija Isasa, M. E. *An. Bromatol.*, **28**, 341 (1976)
11. Larson, B. L. and Hegarty, H. M. *J. Dairy Sci.*, **60**, 1223 (1977)
12. Ritter, W. *Mitt. Geb. Lebensmittel-unters. Hyg.*, **68**, 240 (1977)
13. Adachi, T., Tanimura, A. and Asahina, M. *J. Vitaminol.*, **9**, 217 (1963)
14. Rogers, L. E. and Porter, F. S. *Pediatrics*, **42**, 423 (1968)
15. Murphey, W. H., Patchen, L. and Guthrie, R. *Biochem. Genet.*, **6**, 51 (1972)
16. Reyes, P. *Anal. Biochem.*, **77**, 362 (1977)
17. Makino, K., Kinoshita, T., Satoh, K. and Sasaki, T. *Nature (London)*, **172**, 914 (1953)
18. Manna, L. and Hauge, S. M. *J. Biol. Chem.*, **202**, 91 (1953)
19. Schwitzer, C. *Biochem. Z.*, **328**, 291 (1956)
20. Beyer, K. H. *Pharm. Ztg.*, **105**, 904 (1960)
21. Trapmann, H. and Devani, M. *Dtsch. Apoth. Ztg.*, **105**, 313 (1965)

22. Rommel, K., Georg, D., Mähr, G. and Török, M. *Med. Welt,* **22,** 1221 (1966)
23. O'Sullivan, W. J. *Aust. N. Z. J. Med.,* **3,** 417 (1973)
24. Marchetti, M., Viviani, R. and Rabbi, A. *Nature (London),* **178,** 805 (1956)
25. Moruzzi, M., Viviani, R. and Marchetti, M. *Biochem. Z.,* **333,** 318 (1960)
26. Marchetti, M., Pasquali, P. and Caldarera, C. M. *Int. Z. Vitaminforsch.,* **36,** 317 (1966)
27. Pasquali, P., Landi, L., Caldarera, C. M. and Marchetti, M. *Biochim. Biophys. Acta,* **158,** 482 (1968)
28. Marchetti, M., Caldarera, C. M. and Moruzzi, G. *Ital. J. Biochem.,* **9,** 378 (1960)
29. Caldarera, C. M., Barbiroli, B., Moruzzi, M. S. and Marchetti, M. *Biochim. Biophys. Acta,* **161,** 156 (1968)
30. Viviani, R., Marchetti, M., Rabbi, A. and Morizzi, G. *Nature (London),* **176,** 464 (1955)
31. Dioguardi, N. and Secchi, G. C. *Acta Vitaminol.,* **11,** 241 (1957)
32. Dolcetta, B. and Massimo, L. *Acta Vitaminol.,* **11,** 257 (1957)
33. Moruzzi, G., Viviani, R., Marchetti, M. and Sanguietti, F. *Nature (London),* **181,** 416 (1958)
34. Villari, V. and Mazzacca, G. *Acta Vitaminol.,* **12,** 69 (1958)
35. Saputo, V. and Nicolis, F. B. *Acta Vitaminol.,* **12,** 328 (1958)
36. Verga, A. *Minerva Pediatr.,* **12,** 1006, (1960)
37. Careddu, P., Appolonio, T. and Cabassa, N. *Acta Vitaminol.,* **14,** 15 (1960)
38. Sansotta, S., Celata, G. and Giorgi, C. *Aggiorn. Pediatr.,* **11,** 363 (1960)
39. Russo, G. and Bonanno, V. *Acta Vitaminol.,* **15,** 61 (1961)
40. Serra, U., Sacchetti, G. and Della Marca, A. *Acta Vitaminol.,* **16,** 193 (1962)
41. Caldarera, C. M. and Marchetti, M. *Nature (London),* **195,** 703 (1962)
42. Marchetti, M., Caldarera, C. M. and Moruzzi, G. *Biochim. Biophys. Acta,* **55,** 218 (1962)
43. Marchetti, M. and Pudu, P. *Arch. Biochem. Biophys.,* **108,** 468 (1964)
44. Caldarera, C. M., Barbiroli, B. and Marchetti, M. *Experientia,* **23,** 521 (1967)
45. Caldarera, C. M., Barbiroli, B. and Marchetti, M. *Nature (London),* **217,** 755 (1968)
46. Sechi, A. M., Borgatti, A. R. and Lenaz, G. *Boll. Soc. Ital. Biol. Sper.,* **44,** 2183 (1968)
47. Viviani, R., Sechi, A. M. and Moruzzi, G. *Int. Z. Vitaminforsch.,* **30,** 95 (1969)
48. Gordonoff, T. and Schneeberger, E. W. *Int. Z. Vitaminforsch.,* **30,** 206 (1959)

49. Shuskevich, S. I., Khalmuradov, A. G. and Shestopalova, V. M. *Vopr. Med. Khim.*, **13**, 136 (1967)
50. Sarma, D. S. R. and Sidransky, H. *J. Nutr.*, **92**, 374 (1967)
51. Monserrat, A. J., Porta, E. A. and Hartcroft, W. S. *Arch. Pathol.*, **87**, 154 (1969)
52. Bunyan, J., Cawthorne, M. A., Diplock, A. T. and Green, J. *Br. J. Nutr.*, **23**, 309 (1969)
53. Sarma, D. S. R., Sidransky, H. *J. Nutr.*, **98**, 33 (1969)
54. Simon, J. B., Scheig, R. and Klatskin, G. *J. Nutr.*, **98**, 188 (1969)
55. Pates, M. M., Buyanovskaya, O. A., Kurkina, V. S., Pavlov, G. T., Pomerantseva, I. I., Tunitskaya, T. A., Turetskaya, I. M. and Tseitsina, A. Y. *Farmakol. Toksikol.*, **32**, 604 (1969)
56. Kotaki, A., Okumura, M., Hasan, S. H. and Yagi, K. *J. Vitaminol.*, **16**, 75 (1970)
57. Davies, T., Kelleher, J., Smith, C. L. and Losowsky, M. S. *Int. J. Vitam. Nutr. Res.*, **41**, 360 (1971)
58. Lipkan, G. N. *Farmakol. Toksikol. (Kiev)*, **7**, 128 (1972)
59. Iwata, H., Kobayashi, K., Suga, Y. and Mochizuki, K. *Vitamins*, **45**, 321 (1972)
60. Cheeke, P. R. *Can. J. Anim. Sci.*, **53**, 165 (1973)
61. Lipkan, G. N. and Maksyutina, N. P. *Farm. Zh. (Kiev)*, **28**, 59 (1973)
62. Egorov, B. B. and Gritsyuk, R. I. *Kosm. Biol. Aviakosmicheskaya. Med.*, **10**, 80 (1976)
63. Balmagiya, T. A., Antonova, G. A. and Khodorova, N. A. *Byull. Eksp. Biol. Med.*, **80**, 18 (1975)
64. Reichard, P. *Adv. Enzymol.* **21**, 263 (1959)
65. Jones, M. E. *Curr. Top. Cell. Regul.*, **6**, 227 (1972)
66. Henderson, J. F. and Paterson, A. R. P. *Nucleotide Metabolisms. An Introduction.*, New York: Academic Press (1973)
67. Raskin, I. In *Vitaminy*, p. 470. Moscow: Meditsina (1974)
68. Howell, R. R. In N. Zöllner and W. Gröbner (eds). *Handbüch der Inneren Medizin*, p. 635. Berlin: Springer (1976)
69. Čihák, A. *Chem. Listy*, **72**, 591 (1978)

2. Pathway of Pyrimidine Synthesis de Novo

Higher organisms and many micro-organisms do not require exogenous pyrimidines and can synthesize pyrimidine nucleotides from simple precursors. In 1944 it became apparent that orotic acid is involved in the synthesis of pyrimidines *de novo* and a few years later it was evident that it is a precursor of nucleic acids [70,71].

The small-molecule precursors of orotic acid were identified by Reichard and Lagerkvist [72]. During *in vitro* incubation, liver slices incorporated labelled ammonia, bicarbonate and aspartate into pyrimidine components of RNA. When the slices were incubated with the labelled precursors in the presence of extracellular orotate, isotopes were found in this extracellular fraction. In this way, orotic acid was recognized as an intermediate in pyrimidine synthesis *de novo*. The labelled orotate was chemically degraded and small molecules identified as the precursors of particular atoms of the orotate ring, as shown in the following scheme:

Nutrition studies in bacteria indicated that carbamoyl aspartate (also known as ureidosuccinate) is an intermediate in pyrimidine biosynthesis. Finally, uridine nucleotides were found as end products of pyrimidine synthesis *de novo* [73]. The sequence of reactions leading to the synthesis of UMP is designated as the orotate pathway or pyrimidine synthesis *de novo* in distinction to the salvage pathway.

The salvage pathway utilizes preformed pyrimidines and purines for the synthesis of nucleic acids and is highly active in various types of cells. Uridine kinase plays a key role in the pyrimidine salvage pathway and its concentration is considered to reflect the relative efficiency of the system in utilizing preformed pyrimidines [74]. Adenosine kinase plays a similar role in making use of preformed purines [75]. It should be noted, however, that uridine and adenosine kinases are not the only enzymes involved in the salvage pathway and other deoxynucleoside kinases, phosphorylases, and phosphoribosyltransferases [76] also have important roles.

As already mentioned, carbamoyl aspartate was recognized as an intermediate in the synthesis of orotic acid [77]. In ureotelic livers, it is synthesized from ammonia, carbon dioxide and aspartic acid in a two-step process, involving the formation of carbamoyl phosphate. When using a rat liver enzyme preparation, ATP and glutamate are necessary for its synthesis. Carbamoyl phosphate is required for the synthesis of urea and arginine, in addition to the synthesis of pyrimidines.

Carbamoyl phosphate synthesis from ammonia represents one of the prominent activities in ureotelic livers [78]. The enzyme requires N-acetylglutamate and is distinct from the enzyme responsible for carbamoyl phosphate synthesis in extrahepatic tissues and in the livers of uricotelic animals. This second enzyme utilizes glutamine [79], rather than ammonia as the primary nitrogen donor and is found in mushrooms, *Escherichia coli*, yeast, Ehrlich ascites tumour and several other animal tissues [80]. This enzyme is carbamoyl phosphate synthetase II (ATP: carbamate phosphotransferase, EC 2.7.2.2) and catalyses the following reaction:

$$\text{Glutamine} + \text{HCO}_3^- + 2\text{ATP} \xrightarrow{\text{K}^+, \text{Mg}^{2+}} \text{glutamate} +$$
$$\text{(or ammonia)} \qquad \text{carbamoyl phosphate} + 2\text{ADP} + \text{P}_i$$

It differs from the Type I enzyme [81] in that both glutamine and ammonia are substrates, although in animal cells glutamine is probably the physiological substrate. A highly active mitochondrial carbamoyl phosphate synthetase I is essential for the detoxication of ammonia through the urea cycle in mammalian livers.

Glutamine-dependent carbamoyl phosphate synthetase II [82,83] is sensitive to allosteric inhibition by UTP and to allosteric activation by 5-phosphoribosyl-1-pyrophosphate (PRPP). Ammonia- and N-acetylglutamate-dependent carbamoyl phosphate synthetase I is neither activated by PRPP nor inhibited by UTP. The sensitivity of the Type II enzyme to feedback inhibition by UTP supports its role in the control of pyrimidine synthesis *de novo*. The enzyme is widely distributed in animal tissues as well as in lower organisms, providing carbamoyl phosphate for pyrimidine biosynthesis [84,85]. The activity of glutamine-dependent synthetase in the tissues is relatively low so it can limit pyrimidine synthesis. Pyrimidine synthesis in the liver *in vivo* is subject to feedback control as can be demonstrated by the immediate stimulation of UMP synthesis by depletion of the end product [86]. A valuable tool in studies of UMP synthesis *de novo* is the depletion of hepatic UTP by D-galactosamine. Using isolated perfused rat livers the concentration of UTP can be reduced in the intact organ to below the normal physiological level [86]. Under these conditions the incorporation of bicarbonate is highly stimulated, providing evidence that glutamine-dependent carbamoyl phosphatase is the site of feedback regulation of liver pyrimidine nucleotide synthesis *in vivo* [87]. Furthermore, the measurement of the rate of incorporation of labelled precursors into orotic acid in slices of various rat tissues demonstrated the operation of a feedback control mechanism

8

governing the rate of pyrimidine synthesis in intact cells and provided evidence that the reaction catalysed by carbamoyl phosphate synthetase II is the site of end product inhibition [88].

Recently a regulatory link has been established between the pathways of pyrimidine and arginine biosynthesis, each of which utilizes carbamoyl phosphate [89]. Orotate exercises an allosteric effect on ornithine transcarbamylase and this effect is dependent upon both the carbamoyl phosphate and ornithine concentrations. When the carbamoyl phosphate level is high, orotate has the effect of changing the normally negative co-operativity of ornithine transcarbamylase to a positive one, thus accelerating the conversion of carbamoyl phosphate in the arginine biosynthetic pathway.

When the carbamoyl phosphate level is low, however, orotate only activates the enzyme at low ornithine concentrations and actually causes inhibition when there is a lot of ornithine available. These interactions seem to be designed to achieve the best use of the carbamoyl phosphate, and to ensure that a certain amount is always available for the pyrimidine synthesis pathway. Regulatory interactions between different metabolic pathways are termed as metabolic interlock [90].

During pyrimidine synthesis, carbamoyl phosphate is utilized in a reversible reaction with the equilibrium shifted in favour of the synthesis of carbamoyl aspartate. The reaction is catalysed by aspartate carbamoyltransferase (carbamoyl phosphate: L-aspartate carbamoyltransferase, EC 2.1.3.2) which is widely distributed in nature. Rapidly growing tissues including various tumours are endowed with high levels of this enzyme [91].

Carbamoyl phosphate   Aspartate   Carbamoyl aspartate

Bacterial aspartate carbamoyltransferase is subject to allosteric inhibition [92] by CTP, one of the end products of the pathway. The enzyme from *E. coli* has been extensively studied because of its regulatory properties [92–94]. The native molecule consists of three regulatory subunits and two catalytic ones. However, three different classes of aspartate carbamoyltransferase have been recognized in different bacterial species, differing in molecular size and kinetic properties [95]. The enzyme has also been demonstrated in a number of animal tissues [96] and together with carbamoyl phosphate synthetase II and dihydro-orotase was found in

9

the soluble fraction of cells (in contrast to carbamoyl phosphate synthetase I [78] which takes part in the synthesis of urea and is located in mitochondria).

Although aspartate carbamoyltransferase appears to be a control site in the synthesis of pyrimidines in *E. coli* (and probably other micro-organisms) the corresponding transferase in animal cells does not appear to be a regulatory enzyme. Furthermore, since its activity in various tissues is far greater than that of carbamoyl phosphate synthetase II, animal aspartate carbamoyltransferase is not the rate-limiting enzyme in the pathway.

The conversion of carbamoyl aspartate to orotic acid became evident in work by Lieberman and Kornberg [97] who studied the degradation of orotic acid by an orotate-fermenting bacterium, *Zymobacterium oroticum*, and isolated two intermediates, dihydro-orotate and carbamoyl aspartate. The degradation reactions were found to be reversible and the cell-free extract of *Z. oroticum* converted carbamoyl aspartate back to orotic acid.

The enzyme catalysing the reversible cyclization of carbamoyl aspartate to dihydro-orotate is called dihydro-orotase (L-4,5-dihydro-orotate amino-hydrolase, EC 3.5.2.3). Dihydro-orotase was found in various animal tissues and for the catalytic function requires Zn^{2+} ions [98]. Orotic acid was found to be a competitive inhibitor of dihydro-orotate synthesis though a variety of other pyrimidines had no effect on enzyme activity [99].

The second reaction is catalysed by dihydro-orotate dehydrogenase (L-4,5-dihydro-orotate: oxygen oxidoreductase, EC 1.3.3.1). The enzyme reversibly catalyses the reduction of orotate by NADH and aerobic oxidation of both NADH and dihydro-orotate [100]. Dihydro-orotate dehydrogenase from *Z. oroticum* is a flavoprotein [101] containing FMN, FAD and non-haem iron in a molar ratio 1:1:2. The ferrocyanide–ferricyanide oxidation–reduction couple was found to substitute for oxygen as an intermediate electron carrier in the reduction of cytochrome *c*. Oxygen, therefore, is not an obligatory mediator of the reaction catalysed by dihydro-orotate dehydrogenase [102].

Dihydro-orotate-oxidizing activity in rat liver homogenates can be recovered completely in the mitochondrial fraction [103,104].With the exception of this system all the other enzymes of the orotate pathway appear to be present in the soluble cytosolic fraction. Dihydro-orotate dehydrogenase from rat liver was found to be located on the outer surface of the inner membrane of mitochondria [105]. Dihydro-orotate can diffuse freely from the cytosol into the mitochondria and orotate can diffuse freely from the mitochondria into the cytosol. Therefore no active transport of either dihydro-orotate or orotate is required in pyrimidine synthesis [105]. In addition to inhibiting dihydro-orotase, orotic acid strongly blocks [103] dihydro-orotate oxidation.

However, the activities of enzymes involved in the liver in the early stages of pyrimidine synthesis were found to increase following the administration of a diet supplemented with 1% orotic acid [106]. This has been demonstrated for both aspartate carbamoyltransferase and dihydro-orotase.

The elucidation of the last steps of pyrimidine synthesis *de novo* came from the study of Hurlbert and Potter [107] which showed that uridine nucleotides were intermediates in the conversion of orotate to pyrimidines of nucleic acids. UMP was the first of the three uridine 5'-phosphates to become labelled in this process [108]. The synthesis of UMP from orotate takes place in two steps: the stoichiometric condensation [109] of orotic acid with 5-phosphoribosyl-1-pyrophosphate (PRPP) to form orotidine 5'-phosphate and its subsequent irreversible decarboxylation to UMP:

| Orotate | Orotidine 5'-phosphate | Uridine 5'-phosphate |

The first reaction is catalysed by orotate phosphoribosyltransferase (orotidine 5'-phosphate: pyrophosphate phosphoribosyltransferase, EC 2.4.2.10) which is readily reversible. The equilibrium constant for the forward reaction [109] is about 0.1. The reaction is specific for orotate (the enzyme usually does not accept uracil) and some synthetic analogues of orotic acid (Chapter 6). Orotate phosphoribosyltransferase activity was found in many animal tissues [110] and there are several phosphoribosyl-transferases of broad specifity which are distinct from the enzyme involved in the orotate pathway [111–113].

Orotidylic acid decarboxylase (orotidine 5'-phosphate carboxy-lyase, EC 4.1.1.23) catalyses the only irreversible step in the pyrimidine synthesis *de novo*. The enzyme is competitively inhibited by UMP and CMP [114–116] and some anomalous pyrimidine nucleoside 5'-monophosphates. The activity of orotidylic acid decarboxylase in excess of that of orotate phosphoribosyltransferase accounts for the absence of orotidine 5'-phosphate in the pool of low molecular weight compounds in animal cells.

The cytidine 5'-phosphates do not have an independent pathway of *de novo* synthesis and are derived from uridine 5-phosphates by an amination which occurs at the level of 5'-triphosphates:

$$OMP \rightarrow UMP \rightleftharpoons UDP \rightleftharpoons UTP \rightarrow CTP \rightleftharpoons CDP \rightleftharpoons CMP$$

The reaction requires [117] glutamine, Mg^{2+} ions, and non-stoichiometric amounts of GTP acting as an allosteric effector:

$$UTP + ATP + glutamine \xrightarrow{GTP, Mg^{2+}} CTP + ADP + glutamate + P_i$$

11

There is no evidence for the enzyme deamination of cytidine 5′-phosphates, although deoxycytidylate deaminase is a well known enzyme [118,119]. The direct conversion of cytidine compounds to uridine ones occurs by the deamination of cytidine or cytosine.

References

70. Arvidson, H., Eliasson, N. A., Hammarsten, E., Reichard, P. and von Ubisch, E. *J. Biol. Chem.*, **179**, 169 (1949)
71. Reichard, P. *J. Biol. Chem.*, **197**, 391 (1952)
72. Reichard, P. and Lagerkvist, U. *Acta Chem. Scand.*, **7**, 1207 (1953)
73. Hurlbert, R. B. and Potter, V. R. *J. Biol. Chem.*, **209**, 1 (1954)
74. Čihák, A. and Rada, B. *Neoplasma*, **23**, 233 (1976)
75. Murray, A. W. *Biochem. J.*, **106**, 549 (1968)
76. Blakley, R. L. and Vitols, E. *Ann. Rev. Biochem.*, **37**, 201 (1968)
77. Reichard, P. *Acta Chem. Scand.*, **8**, 795 (1954)
78. Kerson, L. A. and Appel, S. H. *J. Biol. Chem.*, **243**, 4279 (1968)
79. Levenberg, B. *J. Biol. Chem.*, **237**, 2590 (1962)
80. Ito, K. and Uchino, H. *J. Biol. Chem.*, **246**, 4060 (1971)
81. Tatibana, M. and Ito, K. *J. Biol. Chem.*, **244**, 5403 (1969)
82. Tatibana, M. and Shigesada, K. *J. Biochem.*, **72**, 549 (1972)
83. Ishida, H., Mori, M. and Tatibana, M. *Arch. Biochem. Biophys.*, **182**, 258 (1977)
84. Hager, S. E. and Jones, M. E. *J. Biol. Chem.*, **242**, 5674 (1967)
85. Tremblay, G. C., Crandall, D. E., Knott, C. E. and Alfant, M. *Arch. Biochem. Biophys.*, **178**, 264 (1977)
86. Keppler, D., Rudigier, J., Bischoff, E. and Decker, K. *Eur. J. Biochem.*, **17**, 246 (1970)
87. Pausch, J., Wilkening, J., Nowack, J. and Decker, K. *Eur. J. Biochem.*, **53**, 349 (1975)
88. Smith, P. C., Knott, C. E. and Tremblay, G. C. *Biochem. Biophys. Res. Commun.*, **55**, 1141 (1973)
89. Knight, D. M. and Jones, E. E. *J. Biol. Chem.*, **252**, 5928 (1977)
90. Jensen, R. A. *J. Biol. Chem.*, **244**, 2816 (1969)
91. Cohen, P. P. and Marshal, M. *Enzymes*, **6**, 327 (1962)
92. Gerhart, J. C. and Pardee, A. B. *J. Biol. Chem.*, **237**, 891 (1962)
93. Gerhart, J. C. and Schachman, H. *Biochemistry*, **4**, 1054 (1965)
94. Hammes, G. G., Porter, R. W. and Wu, C. W. *Biochemistry*, **9**, 2992 (1970)
95. Prescott, L. M. and Jones, M. E. *Biochemistry*, **19**, 3783 (1970)
96. Lowenstein, J. M. and Cohen, P. P. *J. Biol. Chem.*, **220**, 57 (1956)
97. Lieberman, I. and Kornberg, A. *J. Biol. Chem.*, **207**, 911 (1954)
98. Sander, E. G., Wright, D. L. and McCormick, D. B. *J. Biol. Chem.*, **240**, 3628 (1965)
99. Kennedy, J. *Arch. Biochem. Biophys.*, **160**, 358 (1974)

100. Aleman, V., Handler, P., Balmer, G. and Beinert, H. *J. Biol. Chem.*, **243**, 2560 (1968)
101. Friedmann, H. C. and Vennesland, B. *J. Biol. Chem.*, **235**, 1526 (1960)
102. Miller, R. W. and Kerr, C. T. *J. Biol. Chem.*, **241**, 5597 (1966)
103. Kennedy, J. *Arch. Biochem. Biophys.*, **157**, 369 (1973)
104. Forman, H. J. and Kennedy, J. *Prep. Biochem.*, **7**, 345 (1977)
105. Chen, J.-J. and Jones, M. E. *Arch. Biochem. Biophys.*, **176**, 82 (1976)
106. Bresnick, E., Mayfield, E. D. and Mossé, H. *Mol. Pharmacol.*, **4**, 173 (1968)
107. Hurlbert, R. B. and Potter, V. R. *J. Biol. Chem.*, **195**, 257 (1952)
108. Hurlbert, R. B. and Reichard, P. *Acta Chem. Scand.*, **8**, 701 (1954)
109. Lieberman, I., Kornberg, A. and Simms, E. S. *J. Biol. Chem.*, **215**, 403 (1955)
110. Umezu, K., Amaya, T., Yoshimoto, A. and Tomita, K. *J. Biochem.*, **70**, 249 (1971)
111. Hatfield, D. and Wyngaarden, J. B. *J. Biol. Chem.*, **239**, 2580 (1964)
112. Reyes, P. *Biochemistry*, **8**, 2057 (1969)
113. Kessel, D., Deakon, J., Coffey, B. and Bakamjian, A. *Mol. Pharmacol.*, **8**, 731 (1972)
114. Blair, D. G. R., Stone, J. E. and Potter, V. R. *J. Biol. Chem.*, **235**, 2379 (1960)
115. Creasey, W. A. and Handschumacher, R. E. *J. Biol. Chem.*, **236**, 2058 (1961)
116. Blair, D. G. R. and Potter, V. R. *J. Biol. Chem.*, **236**, 2503 (1961)
117. Long, C. W. and Pardee, A. B. *J. Biol. Chem.*, **242**, 4715 (1967)
118. Scarano, E., Geraci, G., Polzella, A. and Companile, E. *J. Biol. Chem.*, **238**, PC 1556 (1963)
119. Maley, G. F. and Maley, F. *J. Biol. Chem.*, **239**, 1168 (1964)

3. Aggregation of Enzymes of the Orotate Pathway

During purification and heat denaturation experiments the activity of orotidylic acid decarboxylase appears to parallel orotate phosphoribosyl-transferase activity. Also under a variety of physiological conditions both enzymes show closely parallel, co-ordinate changes in activity [120–122]. Orotate phosphoribosyltransferase from murine leukaemia P 1534 J (utilizing as the substrate orotate and 5-fluorouracil) was found to exist as a complex with orotidylic acid decarboxylase (123). Both enzyme activities were eluted together during gel filtration, co-sedimented in sucrose gradients, and remainded associated during salt fractionation. However, they could be separated into a phosphoribosyltransferase and decarboxy-lase component when enzyme preparations previously subjected to limited proteolysis by elastase were sedimented in sucrose gradients [123].

A gene affecting orotate phosphoribosyltransferase and orotidylic acid decarboxylase does not affect a third, metabolically adjacent enzyme, dihydro-orotate dehydrogenase [124]. Both erythrocytes and cultured diploid cell strains from patients with orotic aciduria (Chapter 5) are deficient in orotate phosphoribosyltransferase and/or orotidylic acid decar-boxylase [125]. When mutant homozygous cultures are grown in a medium containing inhibitors of the orotate pathway (5-azaorotate or 6-azauridine), the cells develop nearly normal activity of both enzymes [125,126]. The effect is demonstrable even when the medium contains the product of the pathway (uridine or cytidine) in sufficient amounts to overcome the nutritional requirement imposed on the cells by the inhibitors. However, both drugs do not increase the activity of dihydro-orotate dehydrogenase [124,126]. The pyrimidine pathway is thus subdivided into groups of concurrently responding enzymes.

There are several studies on the effect of allopurinol and its metabolic derivatives on orotate phosphoribosyltransferase and orotidylic acid decar-boxylase [127–129]. The administration of allopurinol to rats results in an increased urinary excretion of orotic acid and orotidine [127,130,131], and in elevated activities of orotate phosphoribosyltransferase and orotidylic acid decarboxylase in erythrocytes [128,129]. Also, in man, the administration of allopurinol and oxipurinol leads to an increase in the specific activity of orotate phosphoribosyltransferase and orotidylic acid decar-boxylase [129]. The enzymes were found to exist in a complex as three different molecular species with molecular weights of 55 000, 80 000 and 113 000 daltons. The larger forms of the complex were more stable than the smaller one. In the presence of allopurinol or oxipurinol ribonucleotides (but not the corresponding free bases) the largest, most stable species predominated [129].

Although allopurinol and oxipurinol are potent inhibitors of UMP synthesis [120,131] through the inhibition of orotidylic acid decarboxylase (oxipurinol with a 2,4-diketo pyrimidine ring is capable of acting as an analogue of orotic acid, and 1-ribosyl-oxipurinol 5′-phosphate [132] is a very effective inhibitor of orotidylic acid decarboxylase) the administration of allopurinol and oxipurinol is followed by an increase of the specific activity of both orotate phosphoribosyltransferase and orotidylic acid decarboxylase [120,127,133]. This effect is attributed to the stabilization of the enzymes [134] or the enzyme complex, the metabolites of allopurinol shifting the complex to a larger and more stable form [129].

There are several reports by Jones and co-workers dealing with the purification, properties and conformation of the orotate phosphoribosyltransferase and orotidylic acid decarboxylase enzyme complex present in mouse Ehrlich ascites cells [135–137]. Multiple molecular forms of orotidylic acid decarboxylase from human erythrocytes and human liver were studied by O'Sullivan and co-workers [138,139]. A bifunctional enzyme complex of orotate phosphoribosyltransferase and orotidylic acid decarboxylase occurs also in mouse liver and brain [140], regardless of the developmental stage of the animal. Both enzyme activities remained co-ordinate in fetal, neonatal, immature and adult liver and brain.

A parallel co-purification similar to that involving the enzymes taking part in the final stages of UMP synthesis *de novo* is found in the case of aspartate carbamoyltransferase with carbamoyl phosphate synthetase in baker's yeast [141]. The two enzyme activities co-eluted from gel filtration on Sepharose 6B together with the feedback site and retained full sensitivity to feedback inhibition by UTP. Analytical ultracentrifugation revealed two major peaks and sucrose gradient centrifugation in the presence of UTP, glutamine and Mg^{2+} ions resulted in co-sedimentation of the two activities and the regulatory site, corresponding to a molecular weight of 800 000 daltons [141]. Omission of glutamine and Mg^{2+} ions from the sucrose gradient caused a distinct peak of carbamoyl phosphate synthetase to trail behind the aspartate carbamoyltransferase. This, together with genetic data [142] supports the view that the gene which controls both enzymes and a regulatory site at which UTP causes feedback inhibition of both activities is a polycistronic operon, coding for the production of two or three polypeptide chains which are associated in a multifunctional aggregate [141].

Five of the enzymes of UMP biosynthesis exist in the soluble fraction of Ehrlich ascites carcinoma as two enzyme complexes [143]. One complex contains the first three enzymes of the pathway, carbamoyl phosphate synthetase, aspartate carbamoyltransferase and dihydro-orotase and has an apparent molecular weight of 800 000 to 850 000 daltons. The second enzyme complex contains orotate phosphoribosyltransferase and orotidylic acid decarboxylase and sediments in a sucrose gradient with 30% dimethyl sulphoxide and 5% glycerol with an apparent molecular weight of 105 000 to 115 000 daltons [143].

Glutamine-dependent carbamoyl phosphate synthetase, aspartate carbamoyltransferase and dihydro-orotase were co-purified as a high molecular weight complex from an extract of unfertilized eggs of *Rana catesbeiana* [144]. UTP was required to maintain the integrity of the complex during the last purification steps and its removal resulted in the dissociation of the complex. Incubation of a mixture of the dissociated enzymes with UTP and Mg^{2+} ions led to their reassociation into the high molecular weight complex.

Similar complexes were observed in rat livers and in other tissues [145–149]. The extensively purified complex of glutamine-dependent carbamoyl phosphate synthetase, aspartate carbamoyltransferase and dihydro-orotase from rat liver had a sedimentation coefficient of 27 S (approximately 900 000 daltons). Treatment of the complex with pancreatic elastase caused a selective inactivation of carbamoyltransferase with concomitant dissociation of the complex [159].

References

120. Fox, R. M., Wood, M. H. and O'Sullivan, W. J. *J. Clin. Invest.*, **50**, 1050 (1971)
121. Pausch, J., Keppler, D. and Decker, K. *Biochim. Biophys. Acta*, **258**, 395 (1972)
122. Hoffman, D. H. and Sweeney, M. J. *Cancer Res.*, **33**, 1109 (1973)
123. Reyes, P. and Guganic, M. E. *J. Biol. Chem.*, **250**, 5097 (1975)
124. Wuu, K.-D. and Krooth, R. S. *Science*, **160**, 539 (1968)
125. Pinsky, L. and Krooth, R. S. *Proc. Natl. Acad. Sci. USA*, **57**, 1267 (1967)
126. Krooth, R. S. *Ann. N.Y. Acad. Sci.*, **179**, 548 (1971)
127. Brown, G. K., Fox, R. M. and O'Sullivan, W. J. *Biochem. Pharmacol.*, **21**, 2469 (1972)
128. Becher, M. A., Argubright, K. F., Fox, R. M. and Seegmiller, J. E. *Mol. Pharmacol.*, **10**, 657 (1974)
129. Gröbner, W. and Kelley, W. N. *Biochem. Pharmacol.*, **24**, 379 (1975)
130. Fox, R. M., Royse-Smith, D. and O'Sullivan, W. J. *Science*, **168**, 861 (1970)
131. Kelley, W. N. and Beardmore, T. D. *Science*, **169**, 388 (1970)
132. Fyfe, J. A., Miller, R. L. and Krenitsky, T. A. *J. Biol. Chem.*, **248**, 3801 (1973)
133. Beardmore, T. D., Cashman, J. S. and Kelley, W. N. *J. Clin. Invest.*, **51**, 1823 (1972)
134. Tax, W. J. M., Veerkamp, J. H., Trijbels, F. J. M. and Schretlen, E. A. M. *Biochem. Pharmacol.*, **25**, 2025 (1976)
135. Kavipurapu, P. R. and Jones, M. E. *J. Biol. Chem.*, **251**, 5589 (1976)
136. Traut, T. W. and Jones, M. E. *J. Biol. Chem.*, **252**, 8374 (1977)
137. Traut, T. W. and Jones, M. E. *Biochem. Pharmacol.*, **26**, 2291 (1977)
138. Brown, G. K., Fox, R. M. and O'Sullivan, W. J. *J. Biol. Chem.*, **250**, 7352 (1975)
139. Campbell, M. T., Gallagher, N. D. and O'Sullivan, W. J. *Biochem. Med.*, **17**, 128 (1977)

140. Reyes, P. and Intress, C. *Life Sci.*, **22**, 577 (1978)
141. Lue, P. F. and Kaplan, J. G. *Can. J. Biochem.*, **49**, 403 (1971)
142. Lacroute, F. *J. Bacteriol.*, **95**, 824 (1968)
143. Shoaf, W. T. and Jones, M. E. *Biochemistry*, **12**, 4039 (1973)
144. Kent, R. J., Lin, R.-L., Sallach, H. J. and Cohen, P. P. *Proc. Natl. Acad. Sci. USA*, **72**, 1712 (1975)
145. Hoogenraad, N. J., Levine, R. L. and Kretchmer, N. *Biochem. Biophys. Res. Commun.*, **44**, 981 (1971)
146. Mori, M. and Tatibana, M. *Biochem. Biophys. Res. Commun.*, **54**, 1525 (1973)
147. Ito, K. and Uchino, H. *J. Biol. Chem.*, **248**, 389 (1973)
148. Mori, M., Ishida, H. and Tatibana, M. *Biochemistry*, **14**, 2622 (1975)
149. Mori, M. and Tatibana, M. *J. Biochem.*, **78**, 239 (1975)

4. Efficiency and Regulation of Pyrimidine Synthesis

There are only a few studies dealing with the cellular uptake of orotic acid. The incorporation of orotic acid into whole cells can be stimulated more than 90-fold by a combination of PRPP and a heat labile factor [150], probably orotate phosphoribosyltransferase. It is assumed [151] that the enzyme attaches to the cell membrane and in the presence of external orotic acid and PRPP leads to the formation of internal orotidine 5'-phosphate. In bacteria the orotate is taken up similarly [151] by a process of group translocation across the membrane involving the participation of orotate phosphoribosyltransferase and requiring PRPP.

On the other hand, there are many reports dealing with the control of pyrimidine biosynthesis [152–154] and especially with the incorporation of orotic acid into RNA and DNA in various biological systems and different experimental conditions [155–176]. The labelled orotic acid was utilized as a useful tool to solve a number of biochemical, pharmacological, physiological, and nutritional problems [177–185]. The degradation of orotic acid is accomplished by a set of reactions which are the reverse of those taking place during the synthesis of orotic acid from low molecular weight precursors. The decarboxylation of orotic acid in some strains of *Mycobacterium*, resulting in the direct formation of uracil was also proposed [186] but this finding awaits further confirmation.

Since the sequence of reactions in the orotate pathway was established mainly in studies with adult rat livers, there are continuing attempts to demonstrate a similar sequence of reactions in other biological systems. For example, the enzymes of the orotate pathway are not very active in fetal rat livers [187]. Orotic acid injected into pregnant females is incorporated to a lesser extent into fetal hepatic RNA than into hepatic RNA of adult rats although the placenta does not block the uptake of orotic acid. However, there is a considerable incorporation of orotic acid on the second day after birth [187] and the specific activity of the weanling rat hepatic RNA attains a superior value to that found in the adult rats. There are several reports dealing with the role of the orotate pathway during development [188–191].

For a long time it has not been known whether the brain itself supplies pyrimidine precursors for the synthesis of RNA *de novo* or whether these precursors must be supplied preformed from extraneural sources. Evidence has been obtained [192] that neural tissue has little capacity for synthesizing pyrimidine nucleotides for its own metabolic needs *de novo*. The incorporation studies in rats suggest that the brain utilizes preformed pyrimidines to a much greater extent than it utilizes the *de novo* pathway. This underlines the importance of the liver and other peripheral organs in the maintenance of normal RNA metabolism of the brain [192], although the brain contains the enzymes of pyrimidine synthesis *de novo* [193,194].

Measurements of the incorporation of labelled bicarbonate into orotic acid established the occurrence of the complete pathway of *de novo* pyrimidine synthesis in rat brain [191]. However, the activity of the orotate pathway is very high in fetal brain and declines rapidly with neural development. The mature rat brain exhibits less than 1% of the activity of the fetal brain at 18 days of gestation. It was supposed that the variation in the ability of the brain to synthesize orotic acid *de novo* is determined by a similar variation in its ability to synthesize carbamoyl phosphate [191].

In avian species a similar question has been investigated, namely, whether the ability to synthesize pyrimidines *de novo* is confined to the liver which may serve as a source of pyrimidines to the extrahepatic tissues, or whether the orotate pathway is active in extrahepatic tissues as well. The data obtained using estrogen-stimulated chick oviduct indicate that extrahepatic tissues of avian species meet their requirements for pyrimidine nucleotides through *de novo* synthesis rather than depending upon the liver or other exogenous sources for a supply of formed pyrimidines [195]. The observation that the rate of pyrimidine synthesis is sensitive to inhibition by purines suggests that the regulation of the biosynthesis of purine and pyrimidine nucleotides might be linked through a common metabolic effect. The data indicate that the reaction catalysed by carbamoyl phosphate synthetase II is the site of this inhibition [195].

Several findings suggest that glutamine-dependent carbamoyl phosphate synthetase and orotate phosphoribosyltransferase are important in the control of UMP synthesis *de novo*. The enzymes have distinct peaks of activity during the S phase of the cell cycle of synchronized HTC cells while very little activity during the G_2 and M phase has been observed [196]. Whereas carbamoyl phosphate synthetase activity increases rapidly during early G_1, orotate phosphoribosyltransferase activity is enhanced only at the late G_1. The stimulated *de novo* pyrimidine synthesis during the S phase serves primarily as a source of nucleotides for RNA synthesis, which reaches a peak during this phase of the cell cycle. In addition, the peak in enzyme levels during the S phase of the cell cycle suggests that both enzymes have a short half-life, their formation is periodic, and the main synthesis takes place during the S phase [196].

Factors responsible for the control of pyrimidine nucleotide synthesis in intact cells have also been investigated using rat hepatoma cells growing in culture [197]. The addition of uridine to the culture medium caused a marked decrease in the rate of *de novo* pyrimidine synthesis. Uridine caused an inhibition of orotate phosphoribosyltransferase and did not affect the activity of carbamoyl phosphate synthetase II, aspartate carbamoyltransferase, dihydro-orotase or orotidylic acid decarboxylase. These findings suggest that in rat hepatoma cells in culture orotate phosphoribosyltransferase might be rate-limiting in the synthesis of UMP [197].

On the other hand, the pattern of an increase of orotate phosphoribosyltransferase activity in regenerating rat livers suggests that the enzyme is not rate-limiting for RNA synthesis at the early stages of liver regeneration [198,199], since the activities of enzymes of the orotate pathway either vary little at the early post-operative stages or increase significantly only many hours after the major changes in RNA synthesis have taken place [200–202].

The results from different laboratories underline the importance of knowledge of the precursor uptake and pools for evaluation of biosynthetic processes [203–206]. Perfused regenerating livers produce 2.5 times as much UMP per gram of liver as do perfused normal livers [205]. However, the absolute amount of orotic acid converted into UMP is higher in perfused normal livers than in regenerating ones. It seems that the levels of total orotic acid uptake and UMP synthesis are similar in intact and regenerating livers of the same size and that the total amount of orotic acid taken up, and the size of the liver are what determine UMP production [205].

At 1 hour after partial hepatectomy there is a 60–100% increase in the capacity of the liver to concentrate [^{3}H]orotate with respect to the radioactivity in plasma [206]. The increase in intracellular radioactivity was already detectable 10 min after operation. The effect of partial hepatectomy on precursor entry was restricted to the liver and has been found to also alter the uptake of thymidine and uridine without any change in the metabolism of orotic acid [206].

A high rate of orotic acid uptake is a common feature of the liver and kidney. However, a transport mechanism for orotic acid is impaired in hepatic neoplasia [207]. Also the uptake of orotate by three transplanted kidney tumours was found to be less than 5% of that in the host kidney cortex [208]. An explanation of the decrease in orotate uptake by liver and kidney tumours is not yet known.

References

150. Miyamoto, M. and Terayama, H. *Biochim. Biophys. Acta,* **272,** 612 (1972)
151. Hochstadt, J. *Crit. Rev. Biochem.,* **2,** 259 (1974)
152. Krooth, R. S. *Symp. Int. Soc. Cell. Biol.,* **9,** 43 (1971)
153. Pausch, J. and Decker, K. *Digestion,* **8,** 138 (1973)
154. Smith, P. C., Knott, C. E. and Tremblay, G. C. *Biochem. Biophys. Res. Commun.,* **55,** 1141 (1973)
155. Schneider, J. H. *Biochim. Biophys. Acta,* **51,** 60 (1961)
156. Egyhazi, E. and Hydén, H. *Life Sci.,* **5,** 1215 (1966)
157. Avdalovič, N. *Biochem. J.,* **119,** 331 (1970)
158. Yu, F.-L. and Feigelson, P. *Arch. Biochem. Biophys.,* **141,** 662 (1970)
159. Popov, N., Schmidt, S., Schulzeck, S. and Matthies, H. *Acta Biol. Med. Ger.,* **28,** 13 (1972)
160. Ekren, T. and Yatvin, M. B. *Biochim. Biophys. Acta,* **281,** 263 (1972)
161. Chandler, A. M. and Johnson, L. R. *Proc. Soc. Exp. Biol. Med.,* **141,** 110 (1972)

162. Kochakian, C. D., Dubovsky, J. and Broulik, P. *Endocrinology*, **90**, 531 (1972)
163. Archer, S. J. and Wust, C. J. *Proc. Soc. Exp. Biol. Med.*, **142**, 262 (1973)
164. Cihák, A., Garret, C. and Pitot, H. C. *Eur. J. Biochem.*, **34**, 68 (1974)
165. Pfeifer, G. D. and Szepesi, B. *J. Nutr.*, **104**, 1178 (1974)
166. Casagrande, A., Lazzarini, G., Amore, R. and Cupello, A. *Boll. Soc. Ital. Biol. Sper.*, **50**, 1941 (1974)
167. Glazer, R. I., Nutter, R. C., Glass, L. E. and Menger, F. M. *Cancer Res.*, **34**, 2451 (1974)
168. Markov. G. G., Dessev, G. N., Russev, G. C. and Tsanev, R. G. *Biochem. J.*, **146**, 41 (1975)
169. Villela, G. G. and Jansen, S. *Rev. Bras. Biol.*, **35**, 509 (1975)
170. Lewan, L., Petersen, I. and Yngner, T. *Z. Physiol. Chem.*, **356**, 425 (1975)
171. Yngner, T., Lewan, L. and Petersen, I. *Experientia*, **31**, 387 (1975)
172. Ohnuma, T., Roboz, J., Shapiro, M. L. and Holland, J. F. *Cancer Res.*, **37**, 2043 (1977)
173. Engelbrecht, C., Lewan, L. and Yngner, T. *Experientia*, **33**, 302 (1977)
174. Alam, S. N. and Shires, T. K. *Biochem. Biophys. Res. Commun.*, **74**, 1441 (1977)
175. Glazer, R. I. *Biochim. Biophys. Acta*, **475**, 492 (1977)
176. Bushnell, D. E. and Jeter, J. R. *Cancer Res.*, **38**, 2533 (1978)
177. Shafritz, D. A. and Senior, J. R. *Biochim. Biophys. Acta*, **141**, 332 (1967)
178. Aonuma, S., Hama, T., Tamaki, N. and Okumura, H. *J. Biochem.*, **66**, 123 (1969)
179. Matsushita, S. and Fauburg, B. L. *Circ. Res.*, **27**, 415 (1970)
180. Gomez, O. J., Duvilanski, B. H., Soto, A. M. and Guglielmone, A. F. *Brain Res.*, **44**, 231 (1972)
181. Dewar, A. J. and Winterburn, A. K. *J. Neurol. Sci.*, **20**, 279 (1973)
182. Yoneda, S., Carvalho, R. P. S. and Castellani, B. R. *Rev. Inst. Med. Trop. Sao Paulo*, **16**, 328 (1974)
183. Robinson, J. L. and Larson, B. L. *J. Dairy Sci.*, **57**, 1410 (1974)
184. Fausto, N., Brandt, J. T. and Kesner, L. *Cancer Res.*, **35**, 397 (1975)
185. Crandall, D. E. and Tremblay, G. C. *Comp. Biochem. Physiol.*, **558**, 571 (1976)
186. Vitols, M. J. Shaposhnikov, V. N., and Shvachkin, J. P. *Dokl. Akad. Nauk SSSR*, **174**, 1202 (1967)
187. Lafarge, C. and Frayssinet, C. *Biochimie*, **54**, 471 (1972)
188. Craddock, V. M. and Magee, P. N. *Biochim. Biophys. Acta*, **134**, 182 (1967)
189. Herbst, J. J., Fortin-Magana, R. and Sunshine, P. *Gastroenterology*, **59**, 240 (1970)

190. Hayashi, T. T. and Macfarlane, K. *Nature (London)*, **246,** 94 (1973)
191. Tremblay, G. C., Jimenez, U. and Crandall, D. E. *J. Neurochem.*, **26,** 57 (1976)
192. Hogans, A. F., Guroff, G. and Udenfriend, S. *J. Neurochem.*, **18,** 1699 (1971)
193. Appel, S. H. *J. Biol. Chem.*, **243,** 3924 (1968)
194. Weichsel, M. E., Hoogenraad, N. J., Levine, R. L. and Kretchmer, N. *Pediatr. Res.*, **6,** 682 (1972)
195. Gulen, S. and Tremblay, G. C. *Arch. Biochem. Biophys.*, **168,** 567 (1975)
196. Mitchell, A. D. and Hoogenraad, N. J. *Exp. Cell Res.*, **93,** 105 (1975)
197. Hoogenraad, N. J. and Lee, D. C. *J. Biol. Chem.*, **249,** 2763 (1974)
198. Fausto, N. *Biochim. Biophys. Acta*, **182,** 66 (1969)
199. Bresnick, E. *J. Biol. Chem.*, **240,** 2550 (1965)
200. Tsukada, K. and Lieberman, I. *J. Biol. Chem.*, **239,** 2952 (1964)
201. Bresnick, E. *Methods Cancer Res.*, **6,** 347 (1971)
202. Čihák, A. and Rabes, H. M. *Neoplasma*, **21,** 497 (1974)
203. Bucher, N. L. R. and Swaffield, M. N. *Biochim. Biophys. Acta*, **108,** 551 (1965)
204. Bucher, N. L. R. and Swaffield, M. N. *Biochim. Biophys. Acta*, **174,** 491 (1969)
205. Fausto, N. *Biochem. J.*, **129,** 811 (1972)
206. Ord, M. G. and Stocken, L. A. *Biochem. J.*, **132,** 47 (1973)
207. Lea, M. A., Bullock, J., Khalil, F. L. and Morris, H. P. *Cancer Res.*, **34,** 3414 (1974)
208. Lea, M. A., Koch, M. R. and Morris, H. P. *Cancer Biochem. Biophys.*, **1,** 265 (1976)

5. Alterations in Orotic Acid Excretion

Enhanced excretion of orotic acid was observed under different physiological [209,210] and nutritional [211–217] conditions. The amount of orotic acid excreted during human pregnancy is about 20–40 mg per day and does not vary substantially during the course of pregnancy [209,210]. Inherited deficiencies of the urea cycle [218], purine nucleoside phosphorylase [219], and especially of orotate phosphoribosyltransferase and orotidylic acid decarboxylase also result in an increased excretion of orotic acid.

In children, deficient levels of ornithine carbamoyitransferase (an enzyme involved in the urea cycle, and which converts ornithine and carbamoyl phosphate to citrulline) [218,220] present as orotic aciduria, a secondary effect resulting indirectly from the accumulation of carbamoyl phosphate. The deficiency of ornithine carbamoyltransferase leads to overall stimulation of pyrimidine synthesis *de novo* which is reflected by an increased production and excretion of orotic acid.

'Classical' orotic aciduria is a rare autosomal recessive disorder which is characterized by retarded growth and excretion of large quantities of orotic acid in the urine [221,222]. The disease was described in 1959 as an inborn error of pyrimidine biosynthesis in patients with crystals of orotic acid in the urine [223]. The urinary excretion of orotic acid by these patients was 1.34 g per day in contrast to approximately 0.014 g per day excreted by normal individuals [222,224]. When the diet of patients was supplemented with uridine, clinical remission and a remarkable reduction in orotic acid excretion took place [221,225,226].

A disorder of pyrimidine excretion somewhat comparable to congenital orotic aciduria [227–229] may be produced (Chapter 6) by the administration of several drugs affecting pyrimidine synthesis *de novo* [230–238].

Orotic aciduria is due to homozygosity for a Mendelian gene affecting the activity of two final enzymes of pyrimidine synthesis *de novo* [239,240]. Individuals homozygous for the mutation are biochemically characterized [210,240] by one of two phenotypes. Type I is most prevalent and exhibits deficient or decreased activity of orotate phosphoribosyltransferase and orotidylic acid decarboxylase while type II is characterized by a deficiency of only the decarboxylase. It was proposed that the deficiency of the two sequential enzyme activities in orotic aciduria is consistent with a defect in a genetic control mechanism [241]. Evidence discovered by Worthy and Kelley [242] suggested, however, that the molecular defect is due to a mutation in a gene that affects the structure of either orotidylic acid decarboxylase or orotate phosphoribosyltransferase and cannot be attributed to a mutation in a regulatory gene.

Orotidylic acid decarboxylase from homozygous mutant cells was found to be more thermostabile and exhibited different electrophoretic mobility when compared to the enzyme from normal cells [243]. Although the differences have been shown for this enzyme only, they could reflect alterations in the primary structure of either orotidylic acid decarboxylase or orotate phosphoribosyltransferase since they exist in a complex. Moreover, orotidylic acid decarboxylase itself may be composed of subunits which are in dynamic equilibrium with the aggregate form [244].

References

209. Wood, M. H. and O'Sullivan, W. J. *Am. J. Obstet. Gynecol.*, **116**, 57 (1973)
210. Fox, R. M., Wood, M. H., Royse-Smith, D. and O'Sullivan, W. J. *Am. J. Med.*, **55**, 791 (1973)
211. Kesner, L. *J. Biol. Chem.*, **240**, 1722 (1965)
212. Caraceni, O., Marugo, M., Scopinaro, N. and Minuto, F. *Boll. Soc. Ital. Biol. Sper.*, **45**, 145 (1969)
213. Milner, J. A. and Visek, W. J. *Nature (London)*, **245**, 211 (1973)
214. Milner, J. A. and Visek, W. J. *Proc. Soc. Exp. Biol. Med.*, **147**, 754 (1974)
215. Milner, J. A., Prior, R. L. and Visek, W. J. *Proc. Soc. Exp. Biol. Med.*, **150**, 282 (1975)
216. Prior, R. L., Milner, J. A. and Visek, W. J. *J. Nutr.*, **105**, 141 (1975)
217. Prior, R. L. and Visek, W. J. *Am. J. Physiol.*, **228**, 828 (1975)
218. Macleod, P., Mackenzie, S. and Scriner, C. R. *Can. Med. Assoc. J.*, **107**, 405 (1972)
219. Cohen, A., Staal, G. E. J., Ammann, A. J. and Martin, D. W. *J. Clin. Invest.*, **60**, 491 (1977)
220. Shih, V. E. and Efron, M. L. In *The Metabolic Basis of Inherited Disease*. J. B. Stanburg, J. B. Wyngaarden and D. S. Fredrickson (eds), p. 370. (McGraw Hill) (1972)
221. Smith, L. H., Sullivan, M. and Huguley, C. M. *J. Clin. Invest.*, **40**, 656 (1961)
222. Becroft, D. M. O. and Phillips, L. I. *Br. Med. J.*, **1**, 547 (1965)
223. Huguley, C. M., Bain, J. A., Rivers, S. L. and Scoggins, R. B. *Blood*, **14**, 615 (1959)
224. Lotz, M., Fallon, H. J. and Smith, L. H. *Nature*, **197**, 194 (1963)
225. Becroft, D. M. O., Phillips, L. I. and Simmonds, A. *J. Pediatr.*, **75**, 885 (1969)
226. Howell, R. R., Klinenberg, J. R. and Krooth, R. S. *John Hopkins Med. J.*, **120**, 81 (1967)
227. Tubergen, D. K., Krooth, R. S. and Heyn, R. M. *Am. J. Dis. Child.*, **118**, 864 (1969)
228. Soutter, G. B., Yu, J. S., Lovric, A. and Stapleton, T. *Aust. Paediatr. J.*, **6**, 47 (1970)
229. Beardmore, T. D. and Kelley, W. N. *Clin. Chem.*, **17**, 795 (1971)
230. Habermann, V. and Šorm, F. *Collect. Czech. Chem. Commun.*, **23**, 2201 (1958)

231. Fallon, H. J., Frei, E., Block, J. and Seegmiller, J. E. *J. Clin. Invest.*, **40**, 1906 (1961)
232. Fallon, H. J., Lotz, M. and Smith, L. H. *Blood*, **20**, 700 (1962)
233. Buttoo, A. S., Israëls, M. C. G. and Wilkinson, J. F. *Br. Med. J.*, **1**, 552 (1965)
234. Zöllner, N. and Gröbner, W. *Z. Gesamte Exp. Med.*, **156**, 317 (1971)
235. Foster, D. M., Lee, C.-S. and O'Sullivan, W. J. *Biochem. Med.*, **7**, 61 (1973)
236. Krooth, R. S., Lam, G. F. M. and Chen Kiang, S. Y. *Cell*, **3**, 55 (1975)
237. Rauch-Janssen, A., Gröbner, W. and Zöllner, N. *Verh. Dtsch. Ges. Inn. Med.*, **82**, 902 (1976)
238. Mangoff, S. C. and Milner, J. A. *Proc. Soc. Exp. Biol. Med.*, **157**, 110 (1978)
239. Krooth, R. S. *Cold Spring Harbor Symp. Quant. Biol.*, **29**, 189 (1964)
240. Fox, R. M., O'Sullivan, W. J. and Firkin, B. G. *Am. J. Med.*, **47**, 332 (1969)
241. Pinsky, L. and Krooth, R. S. *Proc. Natl. Acad. Sci. USA*, **57**, 925 (1967)
242. Worthy, T. E. and Kelley, W. N. *Am. J. Hum. Genet.*, **25**, 880 (1973)
243. Worthy, T. E., Gröbner, W. and Kelley, W. N. *Proc. Natl. Acad. Sci. USA*, **71**, 3031 (1974)
244. Krooth, R. S., Pan, Y.-L. and Pinsky, L. *Biochem. Genet.*, **8**, 133 (1973)

6. Inhibitors of the Orotate Pathway

The first known drug affecting the orotate pathway was 6-azauridine [245,246]. This analogue is phosphorylated to 6-azauridine 5'-monophosphate which acts as a competitive inhibitor of orotidylic acid decarboxylase [247]. Therapeutic use of 6-azauridine [248,249] is occasionally complicated by a pronounced crystalluria. Owing to the block of orotidylic acid decarboxylase, large amounts of orotidine and orotic acid are excreted in urine. After the infusion of 6-azauridine the excretion of orotic acid precedes orotidine and the former disappears more rapidly from the urine. Psoriatic patients on azaribine (triacetylated form of 6-azauridine given orally) excreted 0.2–1.3 g of orotic acid and orotidine per day [250].

The reduction in urinary excretion of both compounds following uridine therapy reflects the utilization of uridine for the formation of UMP by the salvage pathway. A similar phenomenon was observed in hereditary orotic aciduria following uridine replacement therapy which bypasses the congenital enzyme defect (Chapter 5). The reversal of 6-azauridine-induced orotic aciduria by hydroxyurea, methotrexate and cyclophosphamide [251] (i.e. by the drugs affecting the synthesis of DNA without any effect on orotic acid synthesis) suggests that the control of pyrimidine synthesis *de novo* is linked to DNA synthesis.

Murine lymphoma cells in culture exposed to 6-azauridine also accumulate orotic acid and orotidine, but no detectable amount of orotidine 5'-phosphate [252]. In homogenates of the cells the presence of a membrane-bound phosphatase with activity for orotidine 5'-phosphate was demonstrated. When incubated with homogenate the nucleotide was converted to orotidine in the absence of inorganic phosphate, but it was converted to orotic acid in the presence of phosphate, suggesting the presence of orotidine phosphorylase [252].

An inhibitory effect on orotidylic acid decarboxylase was also observed following 5-azacytidine [253,254], another highly active cytostatic agent [253–256]. The direct action of 5-azacytidine 5'-phosphate on enzyme activity *in vitro* has not yet been measured and the evidence for its interaction with the transformation of orotic acid came from the observation that 5-azacytidine increases its urinary excretion in mice [257,258]. The activity of orotidylic acid decarboxylase in liver extracts from 5-azacytidine-treated animals was also decreased in comparison to controls [258].

However, 5-azacytidine displays a dual effect on the uptake of orotic acid into liver RNA. Whereas the short-term treatment resulted in a block of RNA synthesis, the incorporation of orotic acid was extensively increased when 5-azacytidine had been given at longer time intervals before orotic acid [258,259]. A four-fold increase in the uptake of orotic acid into RNA was observed 18–24 hours after 5-azacytidine, without any preferential labelling of individual types of liver RNA. However, since in fasting animals the uptake of orotic acid into liver RNA was enhanced equally and no additional stimulatory effect of 5-azacytidine was observed, it was suggested that the enhanced uptake of orotate into liver RNA reflects the action of the drug on the gastrointestinal tract. This was later confirmed by measuring the effect of 5-azacytidine on gastric secretion [260]. Cycloheximide too, despite having no effect on orotic acid metabolism, enhances the incorporation of orotate into liver RNA [261] and simultaneously depresses gastric secretion [262].

There are several synthetic derivatives of orotic acid and pyrimidine analogues which, after their conversion, interfere with the activity of orotidylic acid decarboxylase [263,264]. While 6-azacytidine 5'-phosphate is only one tenth as active as 6-azauridine 5'-phosphate [265], 5-hydroxyuridine 5'-phosphate [266] and aminouridine 5'-phosphate [267] are potent inhibitors of orotidylic acid decarboxylase. The inhibitory action of allopurinol and of its metabolites on pyrimidine synthesis *de novo* [268] was mentioned in Chapter 3.

5-Fluoro-orotic acid undergoes in the liver the same conversion as orotic acid [269,270]. The 5-fluoro analogue serves as a substrate for orotate phosphoribosyltransferase [270] and the anomalous nucleoside 5'-phosphate so produced inhibits orotidylic acid decarboxylase. A number of 5-substituted orotic acid (5-chloro, 5-bromo, 5-amino, 5-nitro and 5-methyl) analogues were found to be inactive when examined for their ability to react with or inhibit orotate phosphoribosyltransferase [270].

However, 5-fluoro-orotic and orotic acids are utilized differentially for the synthesis of cytoplasmic liver RNA. 5-Fluoro-orotate is incorporated preferentially into a fraction of non-ribosomal RNA which has several properties in common with messenger RNA [271]. Analysis of microsomal RNA showed little or no incorporation of 5-fluoro-orotic acid into either 18 S or 28 S ribosomal RNA. The analogue is rapidly incorporated into 45 S ribosomal precursor RNA but its subsequent processing into mature 18 S and 28 S RNA is inhibited [272]. The analogue also greatly inhibits the incorporation of orotic acid into ribosomal RNA but has little effect on its incorporation into messenger RNA [273].

5-Azaorotic (oxonic) acid represents another analogue of orotic acid with cytostatic activity [274]. The drug inhibits metabolic transformation and incorporation of orotic acid in the liver and kidney [275]. Similarly to 6-azauridine, 5-azacytidine and allopurinol, the administration of 5-azaorotate results in an increased urinary excretion of orotic acid and orotidine [276]. 5-Azaorotate markedly depresses the activity of orotate phosphoribosyltransferase [275,277]. However, an increased level of orotidine 5'-phosphate in the liver of drug-treated animals indicated a polyvalent inhibitory mechanism [278].

By analogy with 5-fluoro-orotate, [270] 5-azaorotate was found to react with PRPP blocking simultaneously and in a competitive manner the phosphoribosyltransferase reaction. The newly formed 5-azaorotate 5'-phosphate and/or 5-azauridine 5'-phosphate then inhibit orotidylic acid decarboxylase [276,278]. The biological effect of 5-azaorotate depends on its metabolic conversion which is different in different target tissues [279,280]. In bacterial systems and L5178Y leukaemia cells the drug is less effective than in the liver or kidney [275]. Dihydro-5-azaorotic acid specifically inhibits dihydro-orotate dehydrogenase [281].

Barbiturates represent another group of inhibitors of the orotate pathway [282,283]. These pyrimidine derivatives affect dihydro-orotate dehydrogenase [284,285]. It was supposed that barbiturates interfere with dehydrogenase activity by binding to flavine coenzymes resulting in the formation of an inactive complex [285]. Amobarbital has been shown to inhibit the incorporation of orotic acid into RNA in exponentially growing cells of *Bacillus cereus* [286] without having any effect on its metabolic conversion. It was found that the drug markedly depressed the uptake of orotate into bacterial cells [286].

A series of other barbiturates (phenobarbital, barbital, thiopental, pentobarbital at 1 mmol l^{-1} concentration inhibit the orotate uptake system without affecting the incorporation of uracil into cellular pyrimidines [287]. While barbituric acid and hexobarbital are less active, phenylethylhydantoin, chlorpromazine and phenethyl alcohol are extremely active. Phenobarbital also depresses the utilization of orotic acid for the synthesis of cytidine nucleotides in the liver [288]. α-Hexachlorocyclohexane, an inhibitor of the phenobarbital type, was even more effective in depressing *de novo* cytidine nucleotide synthesis from orotic acid [289].

References

245. Škoda, J., Hess, V. F. and Šorm, F. *Experientia,* **13,** 150 (1957)
246. Škoda, J. *Handb. Exp. Pharmacol.,* **38/2,** 348 (1975)
247. Handschumacher, R. E. *J. Biol. Chem.,* **235,** 2917 (1960)
248. Handschumacher, R. E., Calabresi, P., Welch, A. D., Bono, V. H., Fallon, H. J. and Frei, E. *Cancer Chemother. Rep.* **21,** 1 (1962)
249. Turner, R. W. and Calabresi, P. *J. Invest. Dermatol.,* **43,** 551 (1964)
250. Milstein, H. G., Cornell, R. C. and Stoughton, R. B. *J. Invest. Dermatol.,* **61,** 183 (1973)
251. Vogler, W. R., Horwitz, S. and Groth, D. P. *Cancer Res.,* **29,** 1371 (1969)
252. Janeway, C. M. and Cha, S. *Cancer Res.,* **37,** 4382 (1977)
253. Čihák, A. *Oncology,* **30,** 405 (1975)
254. Veselý, J. and Čihák, A. *Pharmacol. Ther. Part A,* **2,** 813 (1978)
255. Hrodek, O. and Veselý, J. *Neoplasma,* **18,** 493 (1971)
256. Karon, M., Sieger, L., Leimbrock, S., Finklestein, J. Z., Nesbit, M. E. and Swaney, J. *Blood,* **42,** 359 (1973)
257. Veselý, J., Cihák, A. and Šorm, F. *Biochem. Pharmacol.,* **17,** 519 (1968)
258. Čihák, A. and Brouček, J. *Biochem. Pharmacol.,* **21,** 2497 (1972)

259. Čihák, A., Veselý, J. and Šorm, F. *Collect. Czech. Chem. Commun.,* **38**, 3944 (1973)
260. Korbová, L., Kohout, J. and Čihák, A. *Arch. Int. Pharmacodyn. Ther.,* **209**, 332 (1974)
261. Čihák, A. *Eur. J. Biochem.,* **58**, 3 (1975)
262. Čihák, A., Korbová, L., Kohout, J. and Reutter, W. *Neoplasma,* **25**, 317 (1978)
263. Chelbova, K. V., Golovinsky, E. V. and Hadjiolov, A. A. *Biochem. Pharmacol.,* **19**, 2785 (1970)
264. Kanetti, J. J. and Golovinsky, E. V. *Chem. Biol. Interact.,* **3**, 421 (1971)
265. Handschumacher, R. E., Škoda, J. and Šorm, F. *Collect. Czech. Chem. Commun.,* **28**, 2983 (1963)
266. Smith, D. A. and Visser, D. W. *J. Biol. Chem.,* **240**, 446 (1965)
267. Smith, D. A., Roy-Burman, P. and Visser, D. W. *Biochim. Biophys. Acta,* **119**, 221 (1966)
268. Foster, D. M., Choy-Soong, L. and O'Sullivan, W. J. *Biochem. Med.* **7**, 61 (1973)
269. Stone, J. E. and Potter, V. R. *Cancer Res.,* **17**, 800 (1957)
270. Dahl, J. L., Way, J. L. and Parks, R. E. *J. Biol. Chem.,* **234**, 2998 (1959)
271. Čihák, A., Wilkinson, D. S. and Pitot, H. C. *Adv. Enzyme Regul.,* **9**, 267 (1971)
272. Wilkinson, D. S., Čihák, A. and Pitot, H. C. *J. Biol. Chem.,* **246**, 6418 (1971)
273. Garrett, C. T., Wilkinson, D. S., Tweedle, J. W. and Pitot, H. C. *Arch. Biochem. Biophys.,* **155**, 342 (1973)
274. Granat, P., Creasey, W. A., Calabresi, P. and Handschumacher, R. E. *Clin. Pharmacol. Ther.,* **6**, 436 (1965)
275. Handschumacher, R. E. *Cancer Res.,* **23**, 634 (1963)
276. Čihák, A. and Šorm, F. *Biochim. Biophys. Acta,* **149**, 314 (1967)
277. Rubin, R. J., Reynard, A. and Handschumacher, R. E. *Cancer Res.,* **24**, 1002 (1964)
278. Čihák, A. and Šorm, F. *Collect. Czech. Chem. Commun.,* **33**, 1778(1968)
279. Čihák, A. and Šorm, F. *Biochem. Pharmacol.,* **21**, 607 (1972)
280. Hatfield, P. J., Simmonds, H. A., Cameron, J. S., Jones, A. S. and Cadenhead, A. *Adv. Exp. Med. Biol.,* **41**, 637 (1974)
281. Santilli, V., Škoda, J., Gut, J. and Šorm, F. *Biochim. Biophys. Acta,* **155**, 623 (1968)
282. Mardashev, S. R. and Fitzner, A. B. *Vopr. Med. Khim.,* **13**, 303 (1967)
283. Mandel, H. G., Triester, S. R. and Szapary, D. *Biochem. Pharmacol.,* **19**, 1879 (1970)
284. Fitzner, A. B. *Vopr. Med. Khim.,* **15**, 465 (1969)
285. Fitzner, A. B. and Mardashev, S. R. *Vopr. Med. Khim.* **16**, 99 (1970)

286. Mandel, H. G., Oliver, H. M. and Riis, M. *Mol. Pharmacol.*, **3,** 537 (1967)
287. Mandel, H. G. and Riis, M. *Biochem. Pharmacol.*, **19,** 1867 (1970)
288. Seifert, J. and Vácha, J. *Mol. Pharmacol.*, **9,** 259 (1973)
289. Seifert, J. and Vácha, J. *Drug Metab. Dispos.*, **3,** 430 (1975)

7. Induction of Fatty Liver in Rats

The administration of a purified diet supplemented with 1% orotic acid induces in rats a rapid accumulation of lipids in the liver [290]. Such an effect is species specific and does not seem to occur in humans. The deposition of triglycerides in the liver, accompanied by a decrease in the concentration of plasma lipids, is a common and characteristic feature of fatty liver induced by various drugs. The earliest biochemical change [291,292] detected in rats given orotic acid is an increase in the pool of uridine nucleotides paralleled by a concomitant reduction of the level of adenine nucleotides and the oxidized and reduced forms of NAD.

The fatty infiltration of the liver which accompanies the ingestion of orotic acid does not seem to be accompanied by serious pathological disturbances [293] and is readily reversible, unlike the development of fatty liver induced by a choline deficient diet. Supplementation of the orotic acid diet with adenine essentially modifies the effect of orotic acid [294]. Since PRPP is required for both the synthesis of purines and the metabolism of orotic acid, the decrease in the pool of adenine nucleotides is caused [295,296] by an inhibition of purine synthesis *de novo* due to extensive depletion of PRPP during the conversion of orotic acid to UMP. After the disappearance of orotic acid from the liver of animals previously fed a diet containing orotic acid, stimulation of the synthesis of adenine nucleotides occurred.

Fatty liver developed in rats fed a diet containing orotic acid is characterized by the deposition of droplets of triglycerides in the tubules of the endoplasmic reticulum [297,298]. The reticulum breaks down into individual vesicles which contain lipid droplets 0.2–0.5 μm in diameter which accumulate the apolipoproteins of low and very low density lipoproteins. The liver otherwise appears to be functionally normal, unlike that of animals receiving other lipotrophic agents. The administration of orotic acid has a specific effect on lipoprotein synthesis without overall inhibition of protein synthesis. The effect is selective for hepatic but not intestinal β-lipoprotein production and triglyceride transport [299].

Plasma β-lipoprotein concentration in rats receiving orotic acid falls to less than 1% of normal and rebounds to normal level within 48 hours following withdrawal of orotic acid [300]. When perfused *in situ*, the livers from orotic acid fed rats released α-lipoprotein, albumin, and other plasma proteins but no detectable β-lipoprotein. They also released smaller amounts of cholesterol and phospholipids than normal livers and no triglycerides, although they contained ten times the normal amount of triglycerides [300]. Since β-lipoprotein has a specific role in the normal transport of triglycerides, the fatty liver produced by orotic acid appears to result from the inhibition of synthesis or release of hepatic β-lipoprotein.

Plasma contains an apoprotein which combines with lipids in the liver to form plasma lipoproteins [301]. Rats treated with orotic acid did produce this apoprotein but the formation of plasma lipoproteins from apoprotein

31

is inhibited [302]. Orotic acid thus specifically depresses the formation of the very low density lipoprotein fraction without affecting the synthesis of the protein portion of the lipoprotein. The fat accumulated in the liver is newly synthesized and does not represent fat mobilized from other tissues.

While in rats following the administration of orotic acid the level of acid-soluble purines decreases, it is unaltered in chicks [303]. There is also no apparent increase in lipid concentrations in the liver of chicks after feeding of orotic acid [303,304]. The induction of fatty liver by orotic acid is highly specific; rat is a susceptible animal, but not the chick, mouse or monkey [305].

Concomitant with triglyceride accumulation in the liver of rats receiving orotic acid the liver peroxide content (lipoperoxides and lipohydroperoxides) is increased several times [306]. The alterations in hepatic lipid and nucleotide levels are prevented as well as reversed when an orotic acid-containing diet is supplemented with 0.25% adenine sulphate [294,307], 4-amino-5-imidazolecarboxamide [308] or allopurinol (as little as 0.05% in the diet [309] completely prevents the accumulation of fat in the liver). Beside these compounds several hypolipidaemic drugs are active in preventing triglyceride deposition in association with an increased level of the serum β-lipoprotein [310]. There is a number of reports dealing with the induction and prevention of the orotic acid fatty liver in rats [311–338].

The basic mechanism underlying the pathogenesis of fatty liver is a block in the release of triglycerides into the plasma [300,339]. Since triglycerides are released from the liver into the plasma in the form of lipoproteins the primary defect in fatty liver is either the synthesis or the secretion of lipoproteins, or both.

References

290. Standerfer, S. B. and Handler, P. *Proc. Soc. Exp. Biol. Med.*, **90,** 270 (1955)
291. Creasey, W. A., Hankin, L. and Handschumacher, R. E. *J. Biol. Chem.*, **236,** 2064 (1961)
292. Von Euler, L. H., Rubin, R. J. and Handschumacher, R. E. *J. Biol. Chem.*, **238,** 2464 (1963)
293. Sidransky, H. and Verney, E. *Am. J. Pathol.*, **46,** 1007 (1965)
294. Handschumacher, R. E., Creasey, W. A., Jaffe, J. J., Pasternak, C. A. and Hankin, L. *Proc. Natl. Acad. Sci. USA*, **46,** 178 (1960)
295. Rajalakshmi, S. and Handschumacher, R. E. *Biochim. Biophys. Acta*, **155,** 317 (1968)
296. Kelley, W. N., Fox, J. and Wyngaarden, J. B. *Biochim. Biophys. Acta*, **215,** 512 (1970)
297. Jatlow, P., Adams, W. R. and Handschumacher, R. E. *Am. J. Pathol.*, **47,** 125 (1966)

298. Novikoff, A. B., Roheim, P. S. and Quintana, N. *Lab. Invest.*, **15**, 27 (1966)
299. Windmueller, H. G., Levy, R. I. and Spaeth, A. E. *Adv. Exp. Med. Biol.*, **4**, 365 (1969)
300. Windmueller, H. G. and Levy, R. I. *J. Biol. Chem.*, **242**, 2246 (1967)
301. Roheim, P. S., Miller, L. and Eder, H. A. *J. Biol. Chem.*, **240**, 2994 (1965)
302. Roheim, P. S., Switzer, S., Girard, A. and Eder, H. A. *Biochem. Biophys. Res. Commun.*, **20**, 416 (1965)
303. Bloomfield, R. A., Letter, A. A. and Wilson, R. P. *Biochim. Biophys. Acta,* **187**, 266 (1969)
304. Kruski, A. W. and Narayan, K. A. *Int. J. Biochem.*, **7**, 635 (1976)
305. Valli, E. A., Sarma, D. S. R. and Sarma, P. S. *Indian J. Biochem.*, **5**, 120 (1968)
306. Kinsella, J. E. *Biochim. Biophys. Acta,* **137**, 205 (1967)
307. Windmueller, H. G. *J. Biol. Chem.*, **239**, 530 (1964)
308. Hayano, K., Tsubone, T., Azuma, I. and Yamamura, Y. *J. Biochem.*, **52**, 379 (1962)
309. Windmueller, H. G. and Von Euler, L. H. *Proc. Soc. Exp. Biol. Med.*, **136**, 98 (1971)
310. Elwood, J. C., Richert, D. A. and Westerfeld, W. W. *Biochem. Pharmacol.*, **21**, 1127 (1972)
311. Rajalakshmi, S., Sarma, D. S. R. and Sarma, P. S. *Biochem. J.*, **80**, 375 (1961)
312. Marchetti, M., Puddu, P. and Caldarera, C. M. *Biochem. J.*, **92**, 46 (1964)
313. Windmueller, H. G. and Spaeth, A. E. *J. Biol. Chem.*, **240**, 4398 (1965)
314. Roheim, P. S., Switzer, S., Girard, A. and Eder, H. A. *Lab. Invest.*, **15**, 21 (1966)
315. Klain, G. J. *Biochim. Biophys. Acta,* **144**, 174 (1967)
316. Kinsella, J. E. *Can. J. Biochem.*, **45**, 1206 (1967)
317. Zakim, D. *Fed. Proc. Fed. Am. Soc. Exp. Biol.*, **26**, 412 (1967)
318. Von Euler, L. H. and Windmueller, H. G. *Proc. Soc. Exp. Biol. Med.*, **125**, 1251 (1967)
319. Porta, E. A., Monning, C. and Hartroft, N. S. *Arch. Pathol.*, **86**, 217 (1968)
320. Simon, J. B., Scheig, R. and Klatskin, G. *Proc. Soc. Exp. Biol. Med.*, **129**, 874 (1968)
321. Klain, G. J., Sullivan, F. J. and Meikle, A. W. *J. Nutr.*, **100**, 1431 (1970)
322. Petzold, H., Storch, H. and Hohlfeld, R. *Z. Ges. Inn. Med. Ihre Grenzgeb.*, **25**, 697 (1970)
323. Vaishwanar, I. and Jiddewar, G. G. *Indian J. Biochem.*, **7**, 214 (1970)
324. Torrielli, M. V., Dianzani, M. U. and Ugazio, G. *Life Sci.*, **10**, 99 (1971)

325. Pottenger, L. A. and Getz, G. S. *J. Lipid Res.,* **12,** 450 (1971)
326. Bloom, R. J. and Westerfeld, W. W. *Arch. Biochem. Biophys.,* **145,** 669 (1971)
327. Witting, L. A. *J. Lipid Res.,* **13,** 27 (1972)
328. Hamuro, Y. *Endocrinology,* **90,** 200 (1972)
329. Nassi, P., Cappugi, G., Niccoli, A. and Ramponi, G. *Physiol. Chem. Phys.,* **5,** 109 (1973)
330. Pinelli, A. and Colombo, A. *Riv. Farmacol. Ter.,* **4,** 363 (1973)
331. Feo, C. and Garcon, E. *Biomedicine,* **19,** 61 (1973)
332. Irsigler, K., Flegel, U., Kühn, P. and Schubert, H. *Int. J. Clin. Pharmacol. Ther. Toxicol.,* **8,** 85 (1973)
333. Pottenger, L. A., Frazier, L. E., Dubien, L. H., Getz, G. S. and Wissler, R. W. *Biochem. Biophys. Res. Commun.,* **54,** 770 (1973)
334. Novikoff, P. M., Roheim, P. S., Novikoff, A. B. and Edelstein, D. *Lab. Invest.,* **30,** 732 (1974)
335. Okonkwo, P. O. and Kinsella, J. E. *Experientia,* **30,** 993 (1974)
336. Negishi, I. and Aizawa, Y. *Jap. J. Pharmacol.,* **25,** 345 (1975)
337. Novikoff, P. M. and Edelstein, D. *Lab. Invest.,* **36,** 215 (1977)
338. Sabesin, S. M., Frase, S. and Ragland, J. B. *Lab. Invest.,* **37,** 127 (1977)
339. Rajalakshmi, S., Adams, W. R. and Handschumacher, R. E. *J. Cell. Biol.,* **41,** 625 (1969)

8. Physiological Effects

Increasing experimental evidence indicates an important role of orotic acid in various cellular processes taking place in different types of cells and organisms. Orotic acid has been shown to stimulate the phagocytic activity of leukocytes [340–342] and of the reticuloendothelial system [343] by a process which can be abolished by pretreatment with hydrocortisone. Vitamin B_{12} and folic acid were found to strengthen the normalizing action of orotic acid on the haemopoiesis of animals subjected to a long-term exposure to toxic substances in low dose [344,345]. Orotic acid at a dose of 100 mg/kg body weight suppressed in rats the inhibitory action of thiophosphamide on blood formation [346].

Orotic acid stimulates the healing process. In mice with an experimental injury the daily oral administration of potassium orotate fastened the healing process, the differentiation of fibroblasts, and the formation and transfer of RNA from nucleus to cytoplasm [347]. Also the rate of collagen synthesis was higher during the stimulation of the wound healing process by potassium orotate [348].

The inhibitory effect of orotic acid (and of bovine milk containing orotate) on cholesterol synthesis was observed [349,350]. Orally administered orotic acid decreases the cholesterol level in whole serum and in serum β-lipoproteins, but increases its level in the liver of treated rats [351]. However, orotic acid did not affect the amount of glycolipids and cholesterol in the brain of lysine-deficient rats [352].

In the Soviet Union [353–357], Hungary [358–363], and especially in the German Democratic Republic the action of orotic acid on the central nervous system was studied. Orotic acid was found to affect the nerve cells during regeneration and also the size of the axon [364–366]. The combination of kavain with magnesium orotate prevents the appearance of disturbances in the function of the central nervous system characteristic of sustained hypoglycaemia [358]. There is a therapeutic consequence of this observation for gerontology since in the course of cerebrovascular ageing both the supply of glucose and its catabolism are below the requirements of the brain. Orotic acid was also found to affect functional disturbances in experimental lymphogenic encephalopathy [359] and to protect against neurotoxicity mediated by strychnine [360]. Orotate antagonized absolutely lethal doses of strychnine, with regard to both the prevention of convulsions and to the reduction of mortality.

Magnesium orotate glycinate complex exerts a protective effect on experimental ammonia poisoning [361,362]. In animals stressed neurotoxically by an insecticide carbamate derivative, the administration of magnesium orotate or orotic acid eliminated or lessened the negative reactions caused by the toxin [363]. Significant differences were also found with learning-dull rats, where orotic acid and its magnesium salt facilitated the learning process [367].

The physiological and pharmacological influence of orotic acid on the teaching and memorization processes and the central nervous system generally, was studied by Matthies and co-workers [368–377] and by Rick and co-workers [378]. For the illustration only one finding will be presented. Orotic acid (100 mg/kg bodyweight per day), given intraperitoneally to rats for 14 days before or during elaboration of a conditional visual discrimination, delays the normal extinction of learned behaviour. The length for 50% extinction was 13 days in controls and 215 days in orotic acid treated animals [379].

This effect was inhibited by 6-azauridine [380] which blocks the conversion of orotate to UMP. However, since both UMP and CMP also improve memory extension even in the presence of 6-azauridine, the availability of pyrimidine nucleotides in the brain is likely to be a limiting factor for long-term memory. Orotate does not stimulate relearning directly but results probably in a higher supply of pyrimidine precursors for the increased brain RNA synthesis that occurs during the process (see also 381).

Orotic acid prevents experimental hepatitis induced by D-galactosamine. The experimental hepatitis paralleled by the accumulation of UDP derivatives of D-galactosamine was studied by Decker and co-workers [382–384]. On the basis of ultrastructural and biochemical analyses it was concluded that the liver damage observed after D-galactosamine treatment differs from that seen in human hepatitis in that the former leads to accumulation of liver triglycerides, hyperplasia of the smooth endoplasmic reticulum, and cell necrosis [385,386].

D-Galactosamine causes a trap mechanism which results in a marked decrease of the content of UTP, UDP, UMP, and UDP-sugars which are necessary for the normal synthesis of DNA and RNA in the liver. Pretreatment with orotic acid (and other pyrimidines) causes protection against the deficit of uridine 5'-phosphates, and no hepatitis-like liver damage is induced [387,388]. The galactosamine-induced hepatic injury was also studied following choline orotate [389,390], and later the protective role of orotic acid in drug-induced hepatitis in relation to the age of experimental animals was described [391,392]. The inhibitory action of various drugs on galactosamine-induced hepatitis can be found in the report by Pickering and co-workers [393].

Besides preventing experimental hepatitis, orotic acid displays a protective effect during liver tumorigenesis taking place in the presence of ethionine and some other carcinogens [394] and during carbon tetrachloride intoxication [395–399]. A single oral dose of 25 mg aicamine (4-aminoimidazole-5-carboxamide orotate) per kg administered to rats simultaneously with a subcutaneous injection of 1 ml carbon tetrachloride totally prevented its hepatotoxic effects [400]. Similarly, orotic acid at a dose of 50 mg/kg abolished the carbon tetrachloride-induced changes but failed to normalize the high hepatic content of lipids and triglycerides [400].

Orotic acid and lysine orotate decrease ethanol toxicity [401,402].

Ethanol inhibits (beside other processes) hepatic galactose elimination [403,404] probably owing to a block in UDP-glucose 4' epimerase which is followed by the accumulation of UDP-galactose, trapping of UDP-glucose, and an increase of galactose 1-phosphate concentration [405]. Orotic acid decreases the effect of ethanol by increasing the level of UDP-glucose [405]. The action of orotic acid in relation to experimental galactosaemia and galactose cataract was also investigated [406–408].

The first studies dealing with the effect of orotic acid on the ultrastructure and enzyme level in the liver [409–415], bile secretion [416], liver regeneration [417], and liver glycogen synthesis [418–420] have been performed in the last 10–15 years. Recently, an abnormal metabolism of orotic acid associated with acute hyperammonaemia [421], renal gluconeogenesis in orotic acid fed rats [422], and the action of orotic acid on enchondral ossification [423] have also been studied.

References

340. Chukichev, E. M. *Farmakol. Toksikol.*, **30**, 214 (1967)
341. Pates, M. M. and Buyanovskaya, O. A. *Byull. Eksp. Biol. Med.*, **63**, 76 (1967)
342. Pates, M. M., Belenky, E. E. and Buyanovskaya, O. A. *Byull. Eksp. Biol. Med.*, **68**, 85 (1969)
343. Lazareva, D. N. and Plechev, V. V. *Aktual. Vopr. Allerg. Immun. Zashch. Mekh. Org.*, p. 63 (1973)
344. Pates, M. M. and Buyanovskaya, O. A. *Byull. Eksp. Biol. Med.*, **64**, 27 (1967)
345. Pates, M. M., Buyanovskaya, O. A. and Tunitskaya, T. A. *Farmakol. Toksikol.*, **32**, 729 (1969)
346. Pates, M. M., Belenky, E. E., Pavlov, G. T., Kurkina, V. S., Tunitskaya, T. A. and Turetskaya, I. M. *Farmakol. Toksikol.*, **33**, 355 (1970)
347. Dudnikova, G. N. and Rivnyak, V. V. *Arkh, Patol.*, **38**, 13 (1976)
348. Dudnikova, G. N. *Byull. Eksp. Biol. Med.*, **82**, 1256 (1976)
349. Bernstein, B. A., Richardson, T. and Amundson, C. H. *J. Dairy Sci.*, **59**, 539 (1976)
350. Bernstein, B. A., Richardson, T. and Amundson, C. H. *J. Dairy Sci.*, **60**, 1846 (1977)
351. Yousufzai, S. Y. K. and Siddiqi, M. *Lipids*, **12**, 689 (1977)
352. Lenaz, G., Sechi, A. M. and Borgatti, A. R. *Boll. Soc. Ital. Biol. Sper.*, **44**, 2180 (1968)
353. Meerson, F. Z., Geinisman, I. U. I. A., Larina, V. N., Rozanova, L. S. and Aleksandrovskaya, M. M. *Dokl. Akad. Nauk SSSR*, **174**, 1198 (1967)
354. Dergachev, V. V., Kruglikov, R. L. and Meerson, F. Z. *Byull. Eksp. Biol. Med.*, **63**, 10 (1967)

355. Krauz, V. A. *Farmakol. Toksikol.*, **35**, 537 (1972)
356. Razumova, I. L. and Alekseeva, N. N. *Patol. Fiziol. Eksp. Ter.*, **17**, 76 (1973)
357. Dergachev, V. V., Panchenko, L. F., Lyubimtseva, O. N. and Popicheva, G. E. *Vopr. Med. Khim.*, **19**, 361 (1973)
358. Zoltán, T. Ö. *Acta Gerontol.*, **9**, 525 (1971)
359. Foldi, M., Zoltán, T. Ö. and Gyori, I. Z. *Gerontol.*, **3**, 97 (1970)
360. Zoltán, T. Ö. *Acta Gerontol.*, **2**, 243 (1972)
361. Szelényi, I., Nemesánszky, E., László, G. and Dési, I. *Arzneim. Forsch.*, **21**, 787 (1971)
362. Szelényi, I., Farkas, I., Dési, I. and Nemesánszky, E. *Arzneim. Forsch.*, **21**, 789 (1971)
363. Dési, I., Szelényi, I. and Sós, J. *Arzneim. Forsch.*, **21**, 780 (1971)
364. Brattgård, S.-O., Hydén, H. and Sjöstrand, I. *Nature (London)*, **182**, 801 (1958)
365. Hydén, H. and Pigon, A. *J. Neurochem.*, **6**, 57 (1960)
366. Peterson, A., Bray, J. J. and Austin, L. *J. Neurochem.*, **15**, 741 (1968)
367. Becker-Carus, C. *Arzneim. Forsch.*, **22**, 2067 (1972)
368. Matthies, H. and Lietz, W. *Acta Biol. Med. Ger.*, **19**, 785 (1967)
369. Matthies, H. and Kirschner, M. *Acta Biol. Med. Ger.*, **19**, 789 (1967)
370. Matthies, H. and Lietz, W. *Acta Biol. Med. Ger.*, **19**, 1053 (1967)
371. Ott, T. and Matthies, H. *Acta Biol. Med. Ger.*, **25**, 181 (1970)
372. Loessner, B. and Matthies, H. *Acta Biol. Med. Ger.*, **27**, 221 (1971)
373. Ott, T. and Matthies, H. *Psychopharmacologia*, **20**, 16 (1971)
374. Ott, T. and Matthies, H. *Acta Biol. Med. Ger.*, **26**, 79 (1971)
375. Matthies, H., Fachse, C. and Lietz, W. *Psychopharmacologia*, **20**, 10 (1971)
376. Ott, T. and Matthies, H. *Psychopharmacologia*, **28**, 195 (1973)
377. Krug, M., Ott, T., Schulzeck, K. and Matthies, H. *Psychopharmacologia*, **53**, 73 (1977)
378. Rick, J. T., Oliver, G. W. and Kerkut, G. A. *Q. J. Exp. Psychol.*, **24**, 282 (1972)
379. Matthies, H. *Farmakol. Toksikol.*, **35**, 259 (1972)
380. Ott, T. and Matthies, H. *Psychopharmacologia*, **23**, 272 (1972)
381. Lutz, M. P. and Domino, E. F. *Arch. Int. Pharmacodyn. Ther.*, **211**, 123 (1974)
382. Reutter, W., Lesch, R., Keppler, D. and Decker, K. *Naturwissenschaften*, **55**, 497 (1968)
383. Keppler, D., Lesch, R., Reutter, W. and Decker, K. *Exp. Mol. Pathol.*, **9**, 279 (1968)
384. Decker, K., Keppler, D. and Pausch, J. *Adv. Enzyme Regul.*, **11**, 205 (1973)
385. Meadline, A., Schaffner, F. and Popper, H. *Exp. Mol. Pathol.*, **12**, 201 (1970)
386. Koff, R. S., Gordon, G. and Sabesin, S. M. *Proc. Soc. Exp. Biol. Med.*, **137**, 696 (1971)

387. Keppler, D., Rudigier, J., Reutter, W., Lesch, R. and Decker, K. Hoppe Seyler's *Z. Physiol. Chem.*, **351**, 102 (1970)
388. Decker, K., Keppler, D., Rudigier, J. and Domschke, W. Hoppe Seyler's *Z. Physiol. Chem.*, **352**, 412 (1971)
389. Scharnbeck, H., Schaffner, F., Keppler, D. and Decker, K. *Exp. Mol. Pathol.*, **16**, 33 (1972)
390. Petzold, H. and Neupert, A. *Z. Ges. Inn. Med. Ihre Grenzgeb.*, **27**, 1087 (1972)
391. Platt, D. and Rebscher, R. *Acta Gerontol.*, **3**, 131 (1973)
392. Platt, D., Leinweber, B. and Rebscher, R. *Z. Gerontol.*, **6**, 125 (1973)
393. Pickering, R. W., James, L. G. W. and Parker, F. L. *Arzneim. Forsch.*, **25**, 898 and 1591 (1975)
394. Sidransky, H. and Verney, E. *J. Natl. Cancer Inst.*, **44**, 1201 (1970)
395. Köcher, Z., Habermannová, S., Cerhová, M. and Suva, J. *Acta Vitaminol.*, **6**, 269 (1964)
396. Cartier, P. and Leroux, J.-P. *Rev. Fr. Etud. Clin. Biol.*, **11**, 248 (1966)
397. Kratzsch, K.-H. and Petzold, H. *Ber. Sek. Inn. Med.*, **4**, 284 (1966)
398. Belenky, E. E., Tseitsina, A. Y., Pomerantseva, I. I., Kurkina, V. S., Tunitskaya, T. A. and Soboleva, R. A. *Farmakol. Toksikol.*, **30**, 218 (1967)
399. Pates, M. M., Tseitsina, A. Y., Pomerantseva, I. I., Tunitskaya, T. A. and Turetskaya, I. M. *Farmakol. Toksikol.*, **31**, 717 (1968)
400. Facsar Rab, E., Leszkovszky, G. and Tardos, L. *Acta Pharm. Hung.*, **46**, 57 (1976)
401. Thomas, H. M. *FEBS Lett.*, **7**, 291 (1970)
402. Alvarado-Andrade, R., Munoz, E., Solodkowska, W. and Mardones, J. *Q. J. Stud. Alcohol.*, **33**, 14 (1972)
403. Tygstrup, N., Ranek, L., Ramsøe, K. and Keiding, S. *Alcohol and Aldehyde Metabolizing Systems*. R. G. Thurman, T. Yonetani, J. R. Williamson, B. Chance (eds), p. 469. (Academic Press, New York) (1974)
404. Keiding, S. *Scand. J. Clin. Lab. Invest.*, **34**, 91 (1974)
405. Keiding, S. and Vinterby, A. *Biochem. J.*, **160**, 715 (1976)
406. Gentil, C. *Arch. Franch. Pediatr.*, **21**, 148 (1964)
407. Schrader, K. E., Beneke, G., Rommel, K. and Mähr, G. *Arch. Klin. Exp. Ophthalmol.*, **168**, 358 (1965)
408. Schmidt, B. J., Ramos, A. O., Caldeira, J. A. F. and Monteiro, D. C. M. *J. Pediatr.* **68**, 138 (1966)
409. Kushima, K. *Med. J. Osaka Univ.*, **9**, 549 (1958)
410. Hashimoto, S. *J. Vitaminol.*, **13**, 19 (1967)
411. Holtzman, J. L. and Gillette, J. R. *Biochem. Pharmacol.*, **18**, 1927 (1969)
412. Pidemsky, E. L., Berdinsky, I. S. and Sazonova, V. N. *Farmakol. Toksikol.*, **32**, 167 (1969)

413. Szelényi, I. *Muench. Med. Wochenschr.*, **112**, 1516 (1970)
414. Szelényi, I., Pucsok, J., Nemesánszky, E. and Sós, J. *Arzneim. Forsch.*, **21**, 777 (1971)
415. Nemesánszky, E. and Szelényi, I. *Arzneim. Forsch.*, **21**, 785 (1971)
416. Pidemsky, E. L., Martyusheva, S. M. and Sapko, V. Y. *Patol. Fiziol. Eksp. Ter.*, **15**, 81 (1971)
417. Löw, O., Machnik, G., Arnrich, M. and Urban, J. *Zentralbl. Pharm.*, **113**, 705 (1974)
418. Sůva, J., Cerhová, M., Habermannová, S. and Habermann, V. *Acta Vitaminol.*, **3**, 97 (1961)
419. Sidransky, H., Verney, E. and Wagle, D. S. *Proc. Soc. Exp. Biol. Med.*, **120**, 408 (1965)
420. Sickinger, K., Kattermann, R. and Hannemann, H. *Acta Hepato Splenol.*, **14**, 88 (1967)
421. Statter, M., Russel, A., Abzub-Horowitz, S. and Pinson, A. *Biochem. Med.*, **9**, 1 (1974)
422. Joseph, P. K. and Subrahmanyam, K. *Indian J. Biochem.*, **7**, 261 (1970)
423. Riede, U., Berli, T. and Mihatsch, M. *Beitr. Pathol.*, **149**, 13 (1973)

9. Orotic Acid in Human Therapy

Orotic acid is relatively insoluble compound but some of its salts and derivatives are more soluble and therapeutically highly active [424–432]. The clearance of orotic acid approaches that of creatinine [433], and during drug-induced orotic aciduria it exceeds glomerular filtration [434]. There is evidence that even high doses of orotic acid are not deleterious to human individuals except that they may occasionally obstruct urine flow by forming crystalline deposits [435].

Orotic acid is bound in the serum to proteins [436] and is metabolized in the liver [433]. The binding of orotic acid to serum proteins in children and adults receiving the drug orally at 80 mg/kg bodyweight per day for 28 days was less than 1% [437]. Maximal serum concentrations of orotic acid were attained 2–5 hours after intake and showed great individual variations, ranging from 0.8 to 10 μg per ml. On the other hand, the half-times for disappearance of orotic acid from the serum were about 1 hour and were more uniform [437]. The resorption of orotate was also followed in newborn infants [438], simultaneously with the level of enzyme activities in blood serum [439,440]. In connection with the anti-inflammatory effect of calcium orotate, [441] the calcium and phosphate metabolism in the treated patients was measured [442,443].

Orotic acid at high doses (3–6 g per day) was used with moderate success in adult patients with pernicious anaemia [444]. Kelley and co-workers [445] investigated the use of orotic acid in the treatment of hyperuricaemia. There was a 20–30% inhibition of purine biosynthesis and an increase in renal clearance of uric acid, but orotic acid offered no advantages over other available agents. Orotic acid in combination with vitamin B_{12} was used in children with disturbed memory [446], and in combination with Kanaform in patients with cerebral trauma and vascular affections [447].

In the Soviet Union orotic acid has been studied for a long time in relation to arteriosclerosis, myocardial infarction [449–450] and various cardiopathogenic changes [451–455]. The effect of precursors of nucleic acid synthesis on myocardial contractile function was followed by Zharov and others [456,457]. However, the effect of orotic acid on the development of myocardial hypertrophy was also studied in other countries [458–463].

Orotic acid has been used in the management of neonatal jaundice and of metabolic defects in icterus neonatarum [464–470]. A possible underlying mechanism contributing to the high levels of unconjugated bilirubin in the plasma of premature infants is a transient deficiency in the conjugating ability of the liver, catalyzed by UDP-glucuronyltransferase. Since a contributing factor could be a low level of UDP-glucuronate due to a low production of UMP, the administration of orotic acid and the resulting increase in the level of UMP and uridine coenzymes in the liver might stimulate the conjugation of bilirubin [471]. There appears to be no contraindication for the use of orotic acid for the treatment of hyperbilirubinaemia in premature infants. It is of interest that orotic acid does not have any effect on bilirubin levels in the mature newborn [466].

Kintzel and co-workers [465] achieved lowered levels of bilirubin using 300 mg orotic acid per day. The premature infants subjected to therapy had from the 3rd to the 6th day consistently 25–30% of the earlier serum bilirubin levels. A number of studies related to the effect of orotic acid on bilirubin level in premature infants was carried out under different conditions [472–480]. Recently, the combination of orotic acid with phenobarbital and adenine was tested [481] as a prophylactic preparation against premature hyperbilirubinaemia.

The major attention was devoted to the use of orotic acid, its inorganic salts and organic derivatives for the treatment of chronic and virus hepatitis [482–489] and other forms of liver insufficiency [490–492]. The beneficial effect of orotic acid and other pyrimidine (and purine) precursors of nucleic acids in the liver led to the appearance of several preparations containing orotic acid in combination with vitamins and other components which were used during the treatment of liver insufficiency. There is a number of clinical and experimental data obtained by Wildhirt [489, 496–498], Nieper [441–443], and others [499–506] which show the beneficial role of orotic acid during the treatment of various liver diseases and speak in favour of its therapeutic use.

References

424. Wildhirt, E. *Ther. Umsch.*, **19**, 387 (1962)
425. Zimmer, V. *Arztl. Prax.*, **23**, 3411 (1971)
426. Birkmayer, W. and Rosmanith, H. *Muench. Med. Wochenschr.*, **113**, 387 (1971)
427. Prokop, L. *Wien. Med. Wochenschr.*, **121**, 399 (1971)
428. Hapke, H. J., Sterner, W., Heisler, E. and Brauer, H. *Farmaco*, **26**, 692 (1971)
429. Nieper, H. A. *Z. Praeklin. Geriatr.*, **6**, 127 (1974)
430. Nieper, H. A. *Z. Praeklin. Geriatr.*, **8**, 184 (1974)
431. Nieper, H. A. *Z. Praeklin. Geriatr.*, **9**, 200 (1974)
432. Unarova, S. A. *Dokl. Akad. Nauk Tadzh. SSR.*, **18**, 64 (1975)
433. Weissman, S. M., Eisen, A. Z., Fallon, H., Lewis, M. and Karon, M. *J. Clin. Invest.*, **41**, 1546 (1962)
434. Cardoso, S. S., Calabresi, P. and Handschumacher, R. E. *Cancer Res.*, **21**, 1551 (1961)
435. Smith, L. H., Huguley, C. M. and Bain, J. A. *The Metabolic Basis of Inherited Disease*. J. B. Stanbury, J. B. Wyngaarden and D. S. Fredrickson (eds), p. 1003. (McGraw Hill) (1972)
436. Hinkel, G. K. and Richter, K. *Pädiatr. Grenzgeb.*, **12**, 215 (1973)
437. Walther, H., Meyer, F. P. and Koehler, E. *Zentralbl. Pharm., Pharmakother. Laboratoriumsdiagn.*, **115**, 615 (1976)

438. Hinkel, G. K. and Le Petit, G. *Paediatr. Grenzgeb.*, **12**, 63 (1973)
439. Stomonyakova, S., Novachev, D. and Todorova, K. *Pediatriya (Sofia)*, **15**, 44 (1976)
440. Ivanov, V. R., Ivanova, L. S. and Dubnikova, L. A. *Farmakol. Reparativn. Regener.*, **3**, 68 (1977)
441. Nieper, H. A. *Agressologie*, **10**, 349 (1969)
442. Nieper, H. A. *Agressologie*, **12**, 401 (1971)
443. Nieper, H. A. *Geriatrie*, **4**, 82 (1973)
444. Rundles, R. W. and Brewer, S. S. *Blood*, **13**, 99 (1958)
445. Kelley, W. N., Greene, M. L., Fox, J. H., Rosenbloom, F. M., Levy, R. I. and Seegmiller, J. E. *Metab. Clin. Exp.*, **19**, 1025 (1970)
446. Dergachev, V. V., Pivovarova, G. H., Khamaganova, T. G. and Shaginian, E. V. *Sov. Med.*, **33**, 78 (1970)
447. Wenzel, E. *Wien. Med. Wochenschr.*, **120**, 226 (1971)
448. Ignatjev, M. V. *Kardiologia*, **9**, 91 (1969)
449. Zharov, E. I. *Kardiologia*, **11**, 15 (1971)
450. Simonson, E. and Berman, R. *Am. Heart J.*, **86**, 117 (1973)
451. Pogosova, A. V. and Belenky, E. E. *Vopr. Med. Khim.*, **15**, 343 (1969)
452. Belenky, E. E., Sokolov, I. K., Tunitskaya, T. A. and Teplova, N. P. *Farmakol. Toksikol.* **34**, 472 (1971)
453. Kleimenova, N. N., Alekseeva, S. P. and Belenky, E. E. *Byull. Eksp. Biol. Med.* **75**, 105 (1973)
454. Belenky, E. E., Sokolov, I. K., Lantsberg, L. A., Tunitskaya, T. A. and Kalugina, G. E. *Farmakol. Toksikol.*, **36**, 301 (1973)
455. Nikolaeva, L. F., Cherpachenko, N. M., Veselova, S. A. and Sokolova, R. I. *Circ. Res. Suppl.*, **3**, 202 (1974)
456. Zharov, E. I., Markovskaya, G. I. and Iurasov, V. S. *Kardiologia*, **8**, 59 (1968)
457. Mikunis, R. I. and Morozova, R. Z. *Kardiologia*, **10**, 102 (1970)
458. Villanyi, P., Votin, J. and Rahlfs, V. *Wien. Med. Wochenschr.*, **120**, 76 (1970)
459. Szelényi, I., Sós, J., Rigo, J. and Surtya, M. *Dtsch. Med. J.*, **22**, 1405 and 1409 (1970)
460. Nemesánszky, E., Pavlik, G. and Szelényi, I. *Arzneim. Forsch.*, **21**, 791 (1971)
461. Donohoe, J. A., Williams, J. F., Kolos, G. and Hickie, J. B. *Aust. N. Z. J. Med.*, **4**, 542 (1974)
462. Williams, J. F., Donohoe, J. A., Lykke, A. and Kolos, G. *Aust. N. Z. J. Med.*, **6**, 60 (1976)
463. Mítová, M. and Bednařík, B. *Scr. Med. Fac. Med. Univ. Brun. Purkynianae*, **49**, 259 (1976)
464. Matsuda, I. and Shirahata, T. *Tohoku J. Exp. Med.*, **90**, 133 (1966)
465. Kintzel, H.-W., Hinkel, G. K. and Schwarze, R. *Acta Paediatr. Scand.*, **60**, 1 (1971)
466. Schwarze, R., Kintzel, H.-W. and Hinkel, G. K. *Acta Paediatr. Scand.*, **60**, 705 (1971)

467. Gray, D. W. G. and Mowat, A. P. *Arch. Dis. Child.*, **46**, 123 (1971)
468. Kintzel, H.-W., Braun, W., Hinkel, G. K., Koslowski, H. and Schwarze, R. *Acta Paediatr. Scand.*, **61**, 703 (1972)
469. Hinkel, G. K., Schwarze, R. and Kintzel, H.-W. *Acta Paediatr. Acad. Sci. Hung.*, **13**, 367 (1972)
470. Hinkel, G. K., Schwarze, R. and Kintzel, H.-W. *Schweiz. Med. Wochenschr.*, **102**, 331 (1972)
471. Brodersen, R. *Acta Paediatr. Scand. Suppl.*, **159**, 15 (1965)
472. Beck, K. and Falk, H. *Liver Research.* J. Vandenbroucke, Tijdschrift voor Gastroenterologie, Antwerpen 1967
473. Cachin, M., Alagille, D. *Presse Med.*, **75**, 859 (1967)
474. Hinkel, G. K., Kemmer, C., Kintzel, H.-W., Roschlau, G. and Schwarze, R. *Kinderaerztl. Prax.*, **38**, 247 (1970)
475. Hinkel, G. K., Kintzel, H.-W. and Schwarze, R. *Kinderaerztl. Prax.*, **38**, 323 (1970)
476. Mowat, A. *Arch. Dis. Child.*, **46**, 397 (1971)
477. Hinkel, G. K., Kintzel, H.-W. and Schwarze, R. *Dtsch. Gesundheitwesen*, **27**, 2414 (1972)
478. Krukow, N. and Brodersen, R. *Acta Paediatr. Scand.*, **61**, 697 (1972)
479. Händel, A., Hinkel, G. K., Kintzel, H.-W. and Schwarze, R. *Paediatr. Paedol.* **8**, 307 (1973)
480. Cutillo, S., Meloni, T. and Dore, A. *Acta Paediatr. Scand.*, **63**, 143 (1974)
481. Lindenau, E., Böttcher, M., Bunke, H., Jung, U., Kalz, M., Klinger, W., Weh, L. and Gmyrek, F. *Dtsch. Gesundheitwesen*, **33**, 26 (1978)
482. Rössing, P., Eberhard, H. and Brandenburg, W. *Dtsch. Med. J.*, **7**, 201 (1956)
483. Dotti, F. and Bonetti, G. *Riforma Med.*, **72**, 666 (1958)
486. Baldini, N. *Attual. Diet.* **4**, 20 (1959)
485. Nissen, K. *Landarzt Heft*, **9**, 337 (1961)
486. Kobayashi, K., Tabe, K., Sasaki, I. and Nakamura, T. *Asian Med. J.*, **6**, 1089 (1963)
487. Kubonoya, J., Kimura, M. and Hongo, A. *Asian Med. J.*, **7**, 196 (1964)
488. Yamada, T., Yamaguchi, M., Kuroiwa, S. and Ito, M. *Asian Med. J.*, **8**, 357 (1965)
489. Wildhirt, E. and Selmair, H. *Muench. Med. Wochenschr.*, **109**, 887 (1967)
490. Chanoine, F. *Acta Gastroenterol. Belg.*, **32**, 383 (1969)
491. Riede, U. N., Strässle, H., Bianchi, L. and Rohr, H. P. *Exp. Mol. Pathol.* **15**, 271 (1971)
492. Negret, J. P. *Bordeaux. Med.*, **5**, 973 (1972)
493. Heinrich, H. C. *Med. Welt.*, **35**, 1791 (1966)
494. Heinrich, H. C. *Muench. Med. Wochenschr.*, **110**, 2311 (1968)
495. Heinrich, H. C. *Aerztl. Prax.*, **26**, 65 (1974)
496. Wildhirt, E. *Prax. Kurier*, **12** 10 (1967)

497. Wildhirt, E. *Z. Praktsch. Med.* **83**, 1 (1970)
498. Wildhirt, E. *Informierte Arzt.*, **4**, 18 (1976)
499. Beckmann, K., Brügel, H., Mertz, D. P. *Dtsch. Med. Wöchenschr.*, **81**, 573 (1956)
500. Riemann, D. *Fortschr. Med.*, **32**, 1317 (1970)
501. Rona, L., Doczy, P. and Marros, T. *Aerztl. Prax.*, **22**, 39 (1970)
502. Brunner, G., Vido, I., Perings, E. and Grünwälder, H. *Arch. Pharm.*, **274**, 325 (1972)
503. Wallnöfer, H. *Muench. Med. Wochenschr.*, **114**, 186 (1972)
504. Lie, T. S., Nakano, H., Gappa, P., Böhmer, F. and Ebata, H. *Leber Magen Darm.*, **7**, 361 (1974)
505. Hirsch, W. and Smerlings, H. *Ther. Ggw.*, **115**, 1719 (1976)
506. Ohlen, J. *Prax. Kurier,* **49**, 6 (1977)

Bibliography

A

A1   Ablin, A., Stephens, B. G., Hirata, T., Wilson, K. and Williams, H. E. Nephropathy, xanthinuria and orotic aciduria complicating Burkitt's lymphoma treated with chemotherapy and allopurinol. Metabolism, 21, 771 (1972)

A2   Adachi, T., Tanimura, A. and Asahina, M. A colorimetric determination of orotic acid. J. Vitaminol., 9, 217–226 (1963)

A3   Adams, D. H. Some observations on the incorporation of precursors into ribonucleic acid of rat brain. J. Neurochem., 12, 783–790 (1965)

A4   Alam, S. N. et al. Improved synthesis and mass fragmentometry of 5-fluoroorotic acid. Acta Pharm. Suec., 12, 375–378 (1975)

A5   Alam, S. N. and Shires, Th. K. The labeling of polysomes and rough microsomal membranes by 5-fluoroorotic acid. Biochem. Biophys. Res. Commun., 74(4), 1441–1449 (1977)

A6   Alvarado-Andrade, R., Munoz, E., Solodkowska, W. and Mardones, J. Effects of orotic acid on alcohol consumption and *in vitro* alcohol metabolism in rats. Q.J. Stud. Alcohol, 33, 14–22 (1972)

A7   Amrutavalli, E. and Sarma, P. S. Effect of glucosamine on orotic acid induced fatty liver. Indian J. Biochem. Biophys., 8, 275–277 (1971)

A8   Andersson, J. and Darzynkiewicz, Z. Nucleoprotein changes and uridine incorporation in rat thymus lymphocytes. I. Cellular characterization of age-dependent thymus involution. II. Effect of treatment with anti-thymocyte serum *in vitro*. Exp. Cell Res., 75, 410–416; 417–423 (1972)

A9   Annanurova, L. A. Effect produced by activators of nucleic acid and protein synthesis on adaptation to the intermittent action of high-altitude hypoxia. Farmakol. Toksikol. (Moscow), 37(2), 226–229, (1974) (Russ.)

A10   Aonuma, S., Hama, T., Tamaki, N. and Okumura, H. Orotate as a β-alanine donor for anserine and carnosine biosynthesis and effects of actinomycin D and azauracil on their pathway. J. Biochem., 66(2), 123–132 (1969)

A11   Archer, A. W. The determination of non-fat milk solids in milk bread from the orotic acid content. Analyst, 98, 755–758 (1973)

A12   Archer, St. J. and Wust, C. J. *In vitro* incorporation of orotic acid by spleen and liver cells of rats. Proc. Soc. Exp. Biol. Med., 142, 262–265 (1973)

A13   Arvidson, H., Eliasson, N. A., Hammarsten, E., Reichard, P. and von Ubisch, H. Orotic acid as a precursor of pyrimidines in the rat. J. Biol. Chem., 179, 169–173 (1949)

A14   Ashihara, H. Changes in activities of the *de novo* and salvage pathways of pyrimidine nucleotide biosynthesis during germination of black gram (*Phaseolus mungo*) seeds. Z. Pflanzenphysiol., 81(3), 199–211 (1977)

A15   Avdalovic, N. Disappearance of radioactivity from the various ribonucleic acid pools and acid-soluble fractions of mouse liver and kidney after single injection of labeled orotic acid. Biochem. J., 119(2), 331–338 (1970)

A16   Avdalovic, N. Uptake of radioactive orotic acid and cyclo-leucine into kidneys of normal and castrated mice adapted to a controlled feeding schedule. Bull. Sci. Cons. Acad. Sci. Arts RSF Yougosl. Sect. A, 20(5–6), 146–147 (1975)

A17   Azzena, D., Trasciatti, S. and Capuzzo, R. A clinical trial of aicamin. Minerva Dietol. Gastroent., 23, 345–351 (1977)

B

B1   Bakanova, N. V. and Leutskii, K. M. Effect of orotic acid and vitamin A on the inclusion of $2-^{14}C$-orotic acid into the acid-soluble fraction and nucleic acids of rat tissues. Biol. Nauki (Moscow), 18(2), 61–65 (1975)

B2   Baldini, N. Primi risultati practici dell'impiego dell'acido orotico nella terapia delle epatopatie e delle distrolie infantili. Attual. Diet., 4, 20–23 (1959)

B3   Balmagiya, T. A., Antonova, G. A. and Khodorova, N. A. Mechanisms of the effect of orotic acid on the growth and development of young rats. Bull. Exp. Biol. Med. (Moscow), (3), 18–21 (1975)

B4   Baskin, F., Marsiarz, F. R. and Agranoff, B. W. Effect of various stresses on the incorporation of (3H)-orotic acid into goldfish brain RNA. Brain Res., 39(1), 151–162 (1972)

B5   Beak, B. and Siegel, B. Mechanism of decarboxylation of 1,3-dimethylorotic acid. A possible role for orotate decarboxylase. J. Am. Chem. Soc., 95, 7919–7920 (1973)

B6   Beardmore, T. D. and Kelley, W. N. Ultraviolet-absorbing compounds in urine from patients with hereditary disorders of purine and pyrimidine metabolism. Clin. Chem., 17, 795 (1971)

B7   Beaudry, M. A., Letarte, J., Collu, R., Leboeuf, G., Ducharme, J. R., Melancon, S. B. and Dallaire, L. Chronic hyperammonemia with orotic aciduria. Pyrimidine pathway stimulation. Diabet. Metabol., 1(1), 29–37 (1975)

B8   Beck, K. and Falk, H. Influence of different compounds on glucuronide synthesis and bilirubin elimination. Liver Research, J. Vandenbroucke, Tijdschrift voor Gastroenterologie, Antwerpen, 1967

B9   Becker-Carus, Ch. Einfluß von Magnesium-orotat und Orotsäure auf den Lernprozeß bei der Ratte. Arzneim. Forsch., 22, 2067–2069 (1972)

B10   Beckmann, K., Brügel, H. and Mertz, D. P. Zur Behandlung von Leberparenchymerkrankungen. Erfahrungen mit i.v. Injektionen eines Orotsäure und Purine enthaltenden Präparates. Dtsch. Med. Wochenschr., 81, 573–577 (1956)

B11   Becroft, D. M., Phillips, L. I. and Simmonds, A. Hereditary orotic aciduria: long-term therapy with uridine and a trial of uracil. J. Pediatr., 75, 885–891 (1969)

B12   Belenky, E. E., Tseitsina, A. Y., Pomerantseva, I. I., Kurkina, V. S., Tunitskaya, T. A. and Soboleva, R. A. Vliianie orotovoi kisloty, ee morfolinovoi soli i purinov na sostoianie pecheni pri khronicheskom otravlenii chetyrekhkloristym uglerodom. Farmakol. Toksikol. (Moscow), 30, 218–221 (1967)

B13   Belenky, E. E., Sokolov, I. K., Tunitskaya, T. A. and
       Teplova, N. P. Effect of orotic acid, inosine and some
       purines on the development of cardiac hypertrophy in
       experimental stenosis of the aorta. Farmakol. Toksikol
       (Moscow), 34(4), 472–476 (1971)

B14   Belenky, E. E., Sokolov, I. K., Lantsberg, L. A., Tunits-
       kaya, T. A. and Kalugina, G. E. Prevention of experimental
       epinephrine-induced lesions of the myocardium with potas-
       sium orotate. Farmakol. Toksikol. (Moscow), 36(3), 301–
       304 (1973) (Russ.)

B15   Bellinger, J. F. and Buist, N. R. Rapid column-
       chromatographic measurement of orotic acid. Clin. Chem.,
       17, 1132–1133 (1971)

B16   Benson, P. F. Subribosomal particles in newborn-rat liver.
       Biochem. J., 110, 59P (1968)

B17   Beorot. (Expose über Beorot. Zürich: Queele: Firmenmit-
       teilung Pharmakon A.G.)

B18   Berdinskii, I. S., Pidemskii, E. L. and Sazonova, V. N.
       Effect of orotic acid on some liver functions under normal
       conditions and during experimental hepatitis. Farmakol.
       Toksikol. (Moscow), 32(2), 167–170 (1969) (Russ.)

B19   Bernstein, B. A., Richardson, T. and Amundson, C. H.
       Inhibition of cholesterol biosynthesis by bovine milk, cul-
       tured buttermilk and orotic acid. J. Dairy Sci. 59(3), 539–
       543 (1976)

B20   Bernstein, B. A., Richardson, T. and Amundson, C. H.
       Inhibition of cholesterol biosynthesis and acetyl-coenzyme
       A synthetase by bovine milk and orotic acid. J. Dairy Sci.,
       60(12), 1846–1853 (1977)

B21   Beyer, K.-H. Orotsäure. Ihre Chemie und physiologische
       Bedeutung. Pharm. Zeitung, 105(31), 904–906 (1960)

B22   Bianchi, P. G. and Saccabusi, E. Clinical experience with
       5,4-amino-4,5-imidazolcarboxyamide ureido succinate in the
       management of inflammatory and degenerative liver disease
       and its comparison with an active reference standard. Miner-
       va Gastroenterol., 18(4), 245–256 (1972)

B23   Birkmayer, W. and Rosmanith, H. Verification of gerontotherapeutic effects. (Clinical experimental study on Kava-form.) Münch. Med. Wochenschr. 113, 387–391 (1971)

B24 Blahos, J. New findings on inborn errors of the purine and pyrimidine metabolism. Cas. Lek. Ces., 113, Nr. 39, S. 1177 (1974)

B25 Blattmann, P. and Retey, J. Stereospecificity of the dihydro-orotate-dehydrogenase reaction. Eur. J. Biochem., 30, 130–137 (1972)

B26 Bloom, R. J. and Westerfeld, W. W. The thiobarbituric acid reaction in relation to fatty livers. Arch. Biochem. Biophys., 145, 669–675 (1971)

B27 Bloomfield, R. A., Letter, A. A. and Wilson, R. P. Effect of orotic acid on the lipid and acid-soluble nucleotide concentrations in avian liver. Biochim. Biophys. Acta, 187, 266–268 (1969)

B28 Bock, K. W. Conjugation of bilirubin – enzymatic aspects. Tag. Dtsch. Ges. Inn. Med. Wiesbaden 25–29 (April 1976)

B29 Boctor, A. and Grossman, A. Differential sensitivity of rat liver and rat hepatoma cells to α-amanitin. Biochem. Pharm., 22, 17–28 (1973)

B30 Bode, J. Ch., Zelder, O., Rumpelt, H. J. and Wittkamp, U. Depletion of liver adenosine phosphates and metabolic effects of intravenous infusion of fructose or sorbitol in man and in the rat. Eur. J. Clin. Invest., 3, 436–441 (1973)

B31 Böhles, H. Hyperammoniämie und Orotosäureauss-cheidung bei totaler parenteraler Ernährung in Abhängig-keit von der zugeführten Argininmenge. 3. Internationales Ammoniaksymposium Baden b. Wien, Mai (1977)

B32 Bogenhard, H. Zur Diagnostik und Therapie chronischer Hepatopathien. Erfahrungen mit Orgatract. Ther. Gegenw., 104, 841–853 (1965)

B33 Boncompagni, P. and Rankel, G. Influenza dell'acido oroti-co sull'accrescimento e sul quadro sieroproteico dell'imma-turo. Lattante, 34, 3–7 (1963)

B34 Borodkin, I. U. S. and Krauz, V. A. The role of intracentral and interneuronal relations in the mechanism of short-term memory control. Farmakol. Toksikol. (Moscow) 35, 533–537 (1972) (Russ.)

B35 Borodkin, I. U. S. and Krauz, V. A. Pharmacological analysis of the participation of the hippocampal-reticular complex in memory processes. Zh. Vyssh. Nerv. Deyatel. I. P. Pavlova, 23(1), 166–173 (1973) (Russ.)

B36 Bresnick, E. Studies on the formation of orotic acid by rat liver preparations. Texas Rep. Biol. Med., 21, 505–510 (1963)

B37 Bresnick, E., Mayfield, E. D. and Mossé, H. Increased activity of enzymes for *de novo* pyrimidine biosynthesis after orotic acid administration. Mol. Pharmacol., 4, 173–180 (1968)

B38 Brodersen, R. Metabolic defects in icterus neonatorum. Acta Paediatr. Scand. Suppl., 159, 15 (1965)

B39 Brodersen, R. and Jacobsen, J. On experimental treatment of premature icteric infants with orotic acid. Acta Paediatr. Scand., 60, 362 (1971)

B40 Brown, G. K., Fox, R. M. and O'Sullivan, W. J. Interconversion of different molecular weight forms of human erythrocyte orotidylate decarboxylase. J. Biol. Chem., 250(18), 7352–7358 (1975)

B41 Brown, G. K. and O'Sullivan, W. J. Inhibition of human erythrocyte orotidylate decarboxylase. Biochem. Pharm., 26(20), 1947–1950 (1977)

B42 Brunner, G., Vido, I., Perings, E., Grünwälder, H. Untersuchungen über die Wirkung von Azathioprin, Cholinorotat und Phenobarbital auf Enzyme des endoplasmatischen Reticulum und Mitochondrien der Rattenleber. Naunyn-Schmiedeberg's Arch. Pharmacol., 274, 325–336 (1972)

B43 Bucher, N. L. R. Experimental aspects of hepatic regeneration. N. Engl. J. Med., 277, 686–696; 738–746 (1967)

B44 Bunyan, J., Cawthorne, M. A., Diplock, A. T. and Green, J. Vitamin E and hepatotoxic agents. II. Lipid peroxidation and poisoning with orotic acid, ethanol and thioacetamide in rats. Br. J. Nutr., 23, 309–317 (1969)

B45 Buskirk, J. J. and Kirsch, W. M. Loss of hepatoma ribosomal RNA during warfarin therapy. Biochem. Biophys. Res. Commun., 52, 562–568 (1973)

B46 Buyanovskaya, O. A. Effect of orotic acid on the formation of antibodies during changed reactivity of an organism. Nov. Biokhim. Fiziol. Vitam. Ferment., 17–18 (1972) (C.A. (1973) 51707z)

B47 Byrnes, K. A., Ghidoni, J. J. and Mayfield, E. D. Response of the rat kidney to folic acid administration. I. Biochemical studies. Lab. Invest., 26, 184–190 (1972)

C

C1 Cachin, M. and Alagille, D. Traitement des afféctions hépato-biliaires de l'enfant et de l'adulte par un médicament composé d'acide orotique et de sorbitol. Press. Med., 75, 859–860 (1967)

C2 Caldarera, C. M. and Marchetti, M. Liver ribonuclease and deoxyribonuclease activity of vitamin B_{12}-deficient chicks: effects of orotic acid and methionine. Nature (London), 195, 703–704 (1962)

C3 Caldarera, C. M., Barbiroli, B. and Marchetti, M. [³H] Formate incorporation into liver nucleic acids of chick. Relationships between orotic acid and vitamin B_{12}. Experientia, 23, 521–522 (1967)

C4 Caldarera, C. M., Barbiroli, B. and Marchetti, M. Effect of orotic acid on activity of nuclear DNA-dependent RNA polymerase and polyribosomal profiles in deficient chick liver lacking vitamin B_{12}. Nature (London), 217, 755–756 (1968)

C5 Caldarera, C. M., Barbiroli, B., Moruzzi, M. S. and Marchetti, M. Studies on the effect of orotic acid on nucleic acid metabolism in vitamin B_{12}-deficient chick liver. Biochim. Biophys. Acta, 161, 156–161 (1968)

C6 Campbell, M. T., Gallagher, N. D. and O'Sullivan, W. J. Multiple molecular forms of orotidylate decarboxylase from human liver. Biochem. Med., 17, 128–140 (1977)

C7   Caraceni, O., Marugo, M., Scopinaro, N. and Minuto, F. Orotic acid and hyperuricemia caused by fructose. Boll. Soc. Ital. Biol. Sper., 45, 145–148 (1969) (Ital.)

C8   Cardelli, J., Long, B. and Pitot, H. C. Direct association of messenger RNA labelled in the presence of fluoroorotate with membranes of the endoplasmic reticulum in rat liver. J. Cell Biol., 70, 47–58 (1976)

C9   Cardoso, S. S., Calabresi, P. and Handschuhmacher, R. E. Alterations in human pyrimidine metabolism as a result of therapy with 6-azauridine. Cancer Res., 21, 1551 (1961)

C10   Careddu, P., Appolonio, T. and Cabassa, N. Modificazioni indotte dal cortisone e dell'acido orotico sul quadro istologico e sui processi de coniugazione della bilirubina nell'epatite virale del topo. Acta Vitamin., 14, 15–20 (1960)

C11   Carrella, M., Björkhem, I., Gustafsson, J.-A., Einarsson, K. and Hellström, K. The metabolism of steroids in the fatty liver induced by orotic acid feeding. Biochem. J., 158, 89–95 (1976)

C12   Cartier, P. and Leroux, J.-P. Influence de l'acide inosinique, seul assicié à l'acide orotique, sur les nucléotides libres du foie de rat au cours de l'intoxication tetrachlorée. C. R. Soc. Biol., 158, 1837–1841 (1964)

C13   Cartier, P. and Leroux, J.-P. Influence de l'acide orotique et de l'acide Inosine-monophosphorique sur les nucléotides libres du foie de rats intoxiques par le terachlorure de carbone. Rev. Fr. Etud. Clin. Biol., 11, 248–255 (1966)

C14   Casagrande, A., Lazzarini, G., Amore, R., Cupello, A. and Ferrillo, F. Comparison among various routes of [3H] orotic acid injection for the labeling of brain cortex RNA in the cat. Boll. Soc. Ital. Biol. Sper., 50, 1941–1945 (1974)

C15   Chagovets, R. V., Sushevich, S. I. and Khalmuradov, A. G. Effect of orotic and nicotinic acids on the incorporation of acetate-1-^{14}C in the total lipids and cholesterol of rat liver. Vopr. Pitan., 25, 24–29 (1966) (Russ.)

C16   Chandler, A. M. and Johnson, L. R. Pentagastrin-stimulated incorporation of [^{14}C] orotic acid into RNA of gastric and duodenal mucosa. Proc. Soc. Exp. Biol. Med., 141, 110–113 (1972)

C17   Chanoine, F. Etude clinique l'orotate d'AICA dans les hépatites et les cirrhoses. Acta Gastro-Enterol. Belg., 32, 383–395 (1969)

C18   Charbonnier, A. and Sagon, J. Découverte et étude expérimentale des propriétés cholérétiques de l'acide uracyl-6-carboxylique. Acta Gastro-Enterol. Belg., 27, 295–311 (1964)

C19   Cheeke, P. R. Effects of orotic acid on the development of vitamin E deficiency in rats. Can. J. Anim. Sci., 53, 165–167 (1973)

C20   Chelbova, K. V., Golovinsky, E. V. and Hadjiolov, A. A. The action of some orotic acid analogues on the in vitro incorporation of [^{14}C]-orotate into pyrimidine nucleotides. Biochem. Pharmacol., 19, 2785–2789 (1970)

C21   Chelbova-Khadzhiolova, K. V. Effect of some orotic acid analogues on the incorporation of [^{3}H]-uridine and [^{3}H]-thymidine into RNA and DNA of cultured mouse embryo fibroblasts. Dokl. Bulg. Akad. Nauk, 25, 533–536 (1972)

C22   Chemnitius, K.-H., Machnik, G., Löw, O., Arnrich, M. and Urban, J. Versuche zur medikamentösen Beeinflussung altersbedingter Veränderungen. I. Über die Verminderung des Lipofuscingehaltes in den Ganglienzellen des Nucleus reticularis gigantocellularis von Albinoratten nach Applikation von Centrophenoxin, p-Chlorphenoxyesssigsäure-diäthylaminoäthylesterhydrochlorid und Centrophenoxiorotat. Exp. Pathol., 4, (Suppl.) 163 (1970)

C23   Chen, J.-J. and Jones, M. E. The cellular location of dihydroorotate dehydrogenase: relation to de novo biosynthesis of pyrimidines. Arch. Biochem. Biophys., 176, 82–90 (1976)

C24   Chen, M.-H. and Larson, B. L. Pyrimidine synthesis pathway enzymes and orotic acid in bovine mammary tissue. J. Dairy Sci., 54, 842–846 (1971)

C25   Cheng, C. C. and Roth, B. Pyrimidines of biological and medicinal interest. II. Prog. Med. Chem., 7, 285–341 (1970)

C26   Chou, J. Y. and Dickman, S. R. Effects of urecholine and atropine on canine pancreas slices. On incorporation of adenine and orotic acid into acid-soluble metabolites and RNA. Arch. Biochem. Biophys., 135, 435–450 (1969)

C27   Christopherson, R. I. and Finch, L. R. The assay of orotate by an isotope dilution procedure. Anal. Biochem., 80, 159–167 (1977)

C28   Chukichev, E. M. Vliianie orotata natriiana razvitie asepticheskogo vospaleniia i fagositoz. Farmakol. Toksikol., 30, 214–218 (1967)

C29   Čihák, A., Wilkinson, D. and Pitot, H. C. The effect of pyrimidine analogues and tryptophan on enzyme synthesis and degradation in rat liver. Adv. Enzyme Regul., 9, 267–289 (1970)

C30   Čihák, A. and Šorm, F. Metabolic transformations of 5-azauracil and 5-azaorotic acid in mouse liver and *Escherichia coli*. Effect on the synthesis of pyrimidines. Biochem. Pharmacol., 21, 607–617 (1972)

C31   Čihák, A. and Brouček, J. Dual effect of 5-azacytidine on the synthesis of liver ribonucleic acids. Lack of the relationship between metabolic transformation of orotic acid *in vitro* and its incorporation *in vivo*. Biochem. Pharmacol., 21, 2497–2507 (1972)

C32   Čihák, A., Vesely, J. and Šorm, F. Metabolic alterations of liver regeneration. XI. Modulation of the uptake of orotic acid into ribonucleic acids in regenerating rat liver. Collect. Czech. Chem. Commun., 38, 3944–3951 (1973)

C33   Čihák, A., Lamar, C. Jr. and Pitot, H. C. Studies on the mechanism of the stimulation of tyrosine aminotransferase activity *in vivo* by pyrimidine analogues. The role of enzyme synthesis and degradation. Arch. Biochem. Biophys., 156, 176–187 (1973)

C34   Čihák, A., Garret, Ch. and Pitot, H. C. Labeling of cytoplasmic liver RNA by 6-[^{14}C] orotic and 5-fluoro 2-[^{14}C] orotic acids. Effect of several inhibitors. Eur. J. Biochem., 34, 68–76 (1973)

C35   Cohen, A., Staal, G. E. J., Ammann, J. A. and Martin, D. W. Jr. Orotic aciduria in two unrelated patients with inherited deficiencies of purine nucleoside phosphorylase. J. Clin. Invest., 60, 491–494 (1977)

C36 Combs, G. F., Arscott, G. H. and Jones, H. L. Unidentified growth factors required by chicks and poults. III. Chick studies involving practical-type rations. Poult. Sci., 33, 77–83 (1954)

C37 Cox, R., Martin, J. T. and Shinozuka, H. Studies on acute methionine toxicity. II. Inhibition of ribonucleic acid synthesis in guinea pig liver by methionine and ethionine. Lab. Invest., 29, 54–59 (1973)

C38 Craddock, V. M. and Magee, P. N. The conservation of isotopically labelled formate and orotate after administration to neonatal animals. Biochim. Biophys. Acta, 134, 182–184 (1967)

C39 Crandall, D. E., Lovatt, C. J. and Tremblay, G. C. Regulation of pyrimidine biosynthesis by purine and pyrimidine nucleosides in slices of rat tissues. Arch. Biochem. Biophys., 188, 194–205 (1978)

C40 Creasey, W. A., Hankin, L. and Handschuhmacher, R. E. Fatty livers induced by orotic acid. I. Accumulation and metabolism of lipids. J. Biol. Chem., 236, 2064–2070 (1961)

C41 Cutillo, S., Meloni, T. and Dore, A. Effect of orotic acid upon serum bilirubin in newborn infants with erythrocyte G-6-PD deficiency. Acta Paediatr. Scand., 63, 143–146 (1974)

D

D1 Dallman, P. R. and Manies, E. C. Protein deficiency: contrasting effects on DNA and RNA metabolism in rat liver. J. Nutr., 103, 1311–1318 (1973)

D2 Davies, T., Kelleher, J., Smith, C. L. and Losowsky, M. S. The effect of orotic acid on the absorption, transport and tissue distribution of A-tocopherol in the rat. Int. J. Vitam. Nutr. Res., 41, 360–367 (1971)

D3 Decker, K., Keppler, D., Rudigier, J. and Domschke, W. Cell damage by trapping of biosynthetic intermediates. The role of uracil nucleotides in experimental hepatitis. Hoppe-Seyler's Z. Physiol. Chem., 352, 412–418 (1971)

D4   Decker, K. and Keppler, D. Galactosamine induced liver injury. Progress in liver diseases. Vol. IV, pp. 183–199. New York, Grune and Stratton (1972)

D5   Decker, K., Keppler, D. and Pausch, J. The regulation of pyrimidine nucleotide level and its role in experimental hepatitis. Adv. Enzyme Regul., 11, 205–230 (1973)

D6   Decker, K. and Keppler, D. Galactosamine-induced liver injury. Presented at the Int. Symp. on Hepatotoxicity, March, 25–30 (1973) (Tel Aviv, Israel)

D7   Delbarre, F. and Auscher, C. Traitement de la goutte par l'acide uracil-6-carboxylique et ses dérivés. Presse Méd., 37, 1765–1768 (1963)

D8   Dergachev, V. V., Kruglikov, R. I. and Meerson, F. Z. Vliianie kofaktorov sinteza i predshestvennikov nukleinovykh kislot i belka na formirovanie i sokhranenie oboritelnogo uslovnogo refleksa. Byull. Eksp. Biol. Med., 63, 10–13 (1967)

D9   Dergachev, V. V., Pivovarova, G. N., Khamaganova, T. G. and Shaginian, E. V. Lechenie orotovoi i folievoi kislotami i vitaminom B_{12} detei s narusheniiami pamiatri. Sov. Med., 33, 78–82 (1970)

D10   Dergachev, V. V., Panchenko, L. F., Lyubimtseva, O. N. and Popicheva, G. E. Effect of folic and orotic acids and vitamin B_{12} on the activity of lysomal enzymes in hippocampus and cerebral cortex of rats under training conditions. Vopr. Med. Khim., 19, 361–365 (1973) (Russ.)

D11   Desi, J., Szelenyi, J. and Sos, J. Einfluß von Magnesium-Orotat und Orotsäure auf Lernprozesse gesunder und neurotoxisch geschädigter Ratten. Arzneim. Forsch., 21, 780–785 (1971)

D12   Desi, I., Szelenyi, I. and Sos, J. Restitution der geschädigten Lernvorgänge der Ratten mit Magnesiumorotat und mit Orotsäure. Kiserl. Orvostud., 24, 5–11 (1972)

D13   Dewar, A. J. and Winterburn, A. K. Changes in the incorporation of [^{14}C] orotic acid into brain RNA of visually deprived rats following exposure to light. J. Neurol. Sci. 20, 279–285 (1973)

D14   Dioguardi, N. and Secchi, G. C. Considerazioni sopra
       l'influenza dell'acido orotico sul metabolismo proeico. Acta
       Vitaminol., 11, 241–252 (1957)

D15   Dölle, W., Eisenburg, J., Kuntz, E., Thaler, H. and Wien-
       beck, M. Selecta-Forum über Leber-Therapie Vitamine,
       wenn Hepatitis anhält? Selecta, 23, 2174–2178 (1978)

D16   Dolcetta, B. and Massimo, L. Prime ricerche sull'accres-
       cimento degli immaturi in seguito a somministrazione di
       acido orotico. Acta Vitaminol., 6, 257–260 (1957)

D17   Domschke, W., Keppler, D., Bischoff, E. and Decker, K.
       Cytosine nucleotides in liver. Hoppe-Seyler's Z. Physiol.
       Chem., 352, 275–279 (1971)

D18   Donohoe, J. A., Kolos, G., Williams, J. F. and Hickie, J. B.
       Effects of orotic acid in rats with myocardial hypertrophy.
       IRCS Libr. Compend., 2, 1222 (1974)

D19   Donohoe, J. A., Williams, J. F., Kolos, G. and Hickie, J. B.
       Action of orotic acid as a positive inotropic agent during the
       acute phase of myocardial hypertrophy. Aust. N.Z. J.
       Med., 4, 542–548 (1974)

D20   Dotti, F. and Bonetti, G. Prime esperienze sul trattamento
       delle epatopatie croniche con orotato di potassio. Rif. Med.,
       72, 666–672 (1958)

D21   Dudnikova, G. N. Autoradiographic study of the rate of
       collagen synthesis under conditions which stimulate the
       wound healing process. Byull. Eksp. Biol. Med., 82, 1256–
       1258 (1976) (Russ.)

D22   Dudnikova, G. N. and Ryvnyak, V. V. Autoradiographic
       and electron-microscope study of fibroblasts during stimula-
       tion of the healing process. Arkh. Patol., 38, 13–18 (1976)
       (Russ.)

D23   Dudov, K. P., Dabeva, M. D. and Hadjiolov, A. A.
       Processing and migration of ribosomal ribonucleic acids in
       the nucleolus and nucleoplasm of rat liver nuclei. Biochem.
       J., 171, 375–383 (1978)

D24   Duffaut, M. and Frexinos, J. Effets thérapeutiques de
       l'association acide orotique sorbitol dans le traitement des

ictères. A propos de 30 observations. Rev. Med. Toulouse Suppl., 3, 995–1004

D25 Durschlag, R. P. and Robinson, J. L. Metabolic fate of orotic acid in relation to hepatic fat accumulation. Presented at the 62nd Annual Meeting Atlantic City, New Jersey, April 9–14 (1978) (Abstr.)

E

E1 Easter, R. A. and Baker, D. H. Nitrogen metabolism and reproductive response of gravid swine fed an arginine-free diet during the last 84 days of gestation. J. Nutr., 106, 636–641 (1976)

E2 Edreira, J. G., Hirsch, R. L. and Kennedy, J. A. Production of fatty liver with dietary ethanol despite orotic acid supplementation. Q.J. Stud. Alcohol., 35, 20–25 (1974)

E3 Egorov, B. B. and Gritsyuk, R. J. Effect of orotic acid on the weight dynamics of rats during restricted motor activity. Kosm. Biol. Aviakosmicheskaya Med., 10, 80–82 (1976) (Russ.)

E4 Ekren, T. and Yatvin, M. B. Distribution and incorporation of [^{3}H] orotic acid in free and membrane-bound ribosomes in rat liver after whole body irradiation and prolonged fasting. Biochim. Biophys. Acta, 281, 263–269 (1972)

E5 Elwood, J. C., Richert, D. A. and Westerfeld, W. W. A comparison of hypolipidemic drugs in the prevention of an orotic acid fatty liver. Biochem. Pharmacol., 21, 1127–1134 (1972)

E6 Engelbrecht, C., Lewan, L. and Yngner, T. Serum and liver radioactivity levels in mice after intraperitoneal and subcutaneous injection of [^{14}C] orotic acid. Experientia, 33, 302–304 (1977)

E7 von Euler, L. H., Rubin, R. J. and Handschuhmacher, R. E. Fatty livers induced by orotic acid. II. Changes in nucleotide metabolism. J. Biol. Chem., 238, 2464–2469 (1963)

E8   von Euler, H. L. and Windmueller, H. G. Fatty liver in the rat after intravenous infusion of orotic acid. Proc. Soc. Exp. Biol. Med., 125, 1251–1254 (1967)

F

F1   Facsar Rab, E., Leszkovszky, G. and Tardos, L. The hepatic protecting effect of imidazole derivatives in acute hepatic damage. Acta Pharm. Hung., 46, 57 (1976) (Hung.)

F2   Fallon, H. J., Frei, E., Block, J. and Seegmiller, J. E. The uricosuria and orotic aciduria induced by 6-azauridine. J. Clin. Invest., 40, 1906–1914 (1961)

F3   Fallon, H. J., Lotz, M. and Smith, L. H. Jr. Congenital orotic aciduria: demonstration of an enzyme defect in leukocytes and comparison with drug-induced orotic aciduria. Blood, 20, 700–709 (1962)

F4   Fausto, N. Orotic acid incorporation into cytoplasmic RNA in normal and regenerating liver. Fed. Proc., 26, 624 (1967)

F5   Fausto, N. and van Lancker, J. L. The effect of x-radiation on the incorporation of [^{14}C] orotic acid into rapidly labeled nuclear and cytoplasmic RNA. Arch. Biochem. Biophys., 135, 231 (1969)

F6   Fausto, N. Conversion of orotic acid into uridine 5'-monophosphate by isolated perfused normal and regenerating rat livers. Biochem. J., 129, 811–820 (1972)

F7   Fausto, N., Brandt, J. T. and Kesner, L. Possible interactions between the urea cycle and synthesis of pyrimidines and polyamines in regenerating liver. Cancer Res., 35, 397–404 (1975)

F8   Fedorov, N. A. and Matveenko, V. N. Levels of free pyrimidines and purines in rat liver and incorporation of carbon-14-labeled sodium bicarbonate into these compounds under the action of a single intraperitoneal injection of orotic acid. Vopr. Med. Khim., 17, 260–263 (1971) (Russ.)

F9   Fehér, J., Jakab, L., Tenczer, J. and Szilvási, I. Klinische
      Untersuchungen zur Leberschutzwirkung von 4-Amino-5-
      Imidazolkarboxamid und Orotsäure. Dtsch. Z. Verdau.
      Stoffwechselkr., 37, 175–179 (1977)

F10   Fekete, I. and Tóth, G. Effect of orotic acid on liver
      glycogen of different animal species. Experientia, 32, 332–
      334 (1976)

F11   Fekete, I. Effects of alloxan on orotic acid and glycogen
      content in various vertebrate species. Experientia, 34, 827–
      828 (1978)

F12   Feo, C. and Garcon, E. Steatosis induced in the rat by orotic
      acid. Biomedicine, 19, 61–64 (1973)

F13   Fitsner, A. B. Biosintez orotovoi kisloty v pecheni krys,
      podvergnutykh deistviiu barbituratov. Vopr. Med. Khim.,
      15, 465–467 (1969)

F14   Fitsner, A. B. and Mardashev, S. R. Possible mechanism of
      the inhibitory effect of barbiturate on orotic acid biosynth-
      esis in microscopic sections of rat liver. Vopr. Med. Khim.,
      16, 99–100 (1970) (Russ.)

F15   Foldi, M., Zoltan, O. T. and Gyori, I. Effect of kawain and
      magnesium orotate on functional disturbances in ex-
      perimental lymphogenic encephalopathy. I. Z. Gerontol., 3,
      97–108 (1970) (Germ.)

F16   Forman, H. J. and Kennedy, J. Dihydroorotate-dependent
      superoxide production in rat brain and liver. Arch.
      Biochem. Biophys., 173, 219–224 (1976)

F17   Forman, H. J. and Kennedy, J. Purification of the primary
      dihydroorotate dehydrogenase (oxidase) from rat liver
      mitochondria. Prep. Biochem., 7, 345–355 (1977)

F18   Foster, D. M., Lee, Choy Soong and O'Sullivan, W. J.
      Allopurinol and enzymes of de novo pyrimidine biosyn-
      thesis. Biochem. Med., 7, 61–67 (1973)

F19   Fox, R. M., O'Sullivan, W. J. and Firkin, B. G. Orotic
      aciduria. Differing enzyme patterns. Am. J. Med., 47,
      332–336 (1969)

F20   Fox, R. M., Royse-Smith, D. and O'Sullivan, W. J. Orotidi-
      nuria induced by allopurinol. Science, 168, 861–862 (1970)

F21   Fox, R. M., Wood, M. H. and O'Sullivan, W. J. Coordinate activity and lability of orotidylate phosphoribosyltransferase and decarboxylase in human erythrocytes, and the effects of allopurinol administration. J. Clin Invest., 50, 1050–1060 (1971)

F22   Fox, R. M., Wood, M. H., Royse-Smith, D. and O'Sullivan, W. J. Hereditary orotic aciduria types I and II. Am. J. Med., 55, 791–798 (1973)

F23   Franca, M. do C. de S. and Carneiro Leao, M. de A. Mitotic activity of onion cells grown separately in media containing thalidomide or orotic acid. Mem. Inst. Biocienc., Univ. Fed. Pernambuco, 1, 149–155 (1974)

F24   Fujisawa, K. and Takahashi, T. Interaction of purine and pyrimidine nucleotides in the orotic acid induced fatty liver. Presented at the 5th Sessio Societas Intern. Hepatol., July 12–15 (1968) (Prague/Karlsbad)

F25   Fujisawa, K., Okabe, K. and Takahashi, T. Effect of 4-amino-5-imidazolcarboxamide on experimental liver injury. Asian Med. J., 15, 585–598 (1972)

F26   Fyfe, J. A., Miller, R. and Krenitsky, T. A. Kinetic properties and inhibition of orotidine 5'-phosphate decarboxylase. Effects of some allopurinol metabolites on the enzyme. J. Biol. Chem., 248, 3801–3809 (1973)

G

G1   Galling, G. Incorporation of uridine and of orotate into chloroplast ribosome RNA of Chlorella after treatment with antibiotics. Arch. Mikrobiol., 81, 245–259 (1972) (Germ.)

G2   Gamp, A. Welche Erfahrungen liegen mit Orotsäure und Allopurinol zur Gichtbehandlung vor? Dtsch. Med. Wochenschr., 90, 38 (1965)

G3   Garcia Olmedo, R., Carballido, A. and Torija Isasa, M. E. Orotic acid in milk. An. Bromatol. 28, 341–374 (1976) (Span.)

OROTIC ACID

G4 Garrett, C. T. Effect of 5-fluoroorotic acid administration on the [^{32}P] base composition, DNA–RNA hybridization properties and labeling of polyadenylate-rich RNA in the cytoplasm of rat liver cells. Arch. Biochem. Biophys. 155, 342–354 (1973)

G5 Gentil, C. Etude du métabolisme glucidique au cours de la galactosémie, effet de l'acide orotique sur l'utilisation du galactose. Arch. Fr. Pediatr., 21, 148 (1964)

G6 Glasgow, A. M. and Chase, H. P. Reye's Syndrome. Lancet, 1, 100–101 (1975)

G7 Glazer, R. I. Inhibition by urethan of the synthesis of free and membrane-bound ribosomal RNA in regenerating liver. Cancer Res., 33, 1759–1765 (1973)

G8 Glazer, R. I. Inhibition of the synthesis of nuclear RNA by urethan in regenerating liver. Biochem. Biophys. Res. Commun., 53, 780–786 (1973)

G9 Glazer, R. I., Nutter, R. C., Glass, L. E. and Menger, F. M. 2-Acetylaminofluorene and N-hydroxy-2-acetylaminofluorene inhibition of incorporation of orotic acid-5-[^{3}H] into nuclear ribosomal and heterogeneous RNA in normal and regenerating liver. Cancer Res., 34, 2451–2458 (1974)

G10 Gmyrek, D., Weh, L., Kalz, M., Bunke, B., Cario, W.-R. and Lindeman, E. Zur medikamentösen Prophylaxe der Neugeborenen-Hyperbilirubinämie. 5. Mitteilung: Wirkungssteigerung durch Kombination der Induktoren Phenobarbital und Nikethamid. Dtsch. Gesuntheitwes., 27, 2221–2227 (1972)

G11 Gniwotta, E. and Kirchdorfer, A. M. Behandlung verschiedener Lebererkrankungen mit einem kombinierten Lebertherapeutikum aus essentiellen Aminosäuren, Vitamin B, Folsäure und Nikotinsäureamid. Z. Allgemeinmed./Landarzt 16, 799–802 (1973)

G12 Golovinsky, E., Spassov, A. and Roussinova, E. Effect of some orotaldehyde derivatives as orotic acid antagonists in Neurospora crassa. Z. Naturforsch. Teil B, 24, 1315–1317 (1969) (Germ.)

G13 Golovinsky, E., Kaneti, J., Yukhnovsky, I. and Genchev, D. A study of some orotic acid derivatives and analogues by

66

Huckel's method of molecular orbitals. II. Analogues of the orotic acid in the reaction with phosphoribosyl-pyrophosphate. J. Theor. Biol., 26, 29–32 (1970)

G14   Golovinsky, E., Emanuilov, E. and Markov, G. G. The effect of orotic acid hydrazide on the growth of *Neurospora crassa* and on the development of Ehrlich ascites tumor. Vopr. Med. Khim., 16, 293–295 (1970) (Russ.)

G15   Golovinsky, E. Biochemistry of orotic acid antimetabolites. Hippokrates, 43, 101–103 (1972) (Germ.)

G16   Golovinsky, E. Orotic acid antimetabolites. Vopr. Med. Khim., 18, 451–460 (1972) (Russ.)

G17   Golovinsky, E., Markov, K. and Maneva, L. Effect of some orotic acid derivatives and analogs on the growth of microorganisms. Izv. Inst. Biokhim. Bulg. Akad. Nauk., 4, 17–26 (1973) (Bulg.)

G18   Gomez, O. J., Duvilanski, B. H., Soto, A. M. and Gugliel-mone, A. F. Hormonal regulation of brain development. VI. Kinetic studies of the incorporation *in vivo* of [^{3}H] orotic acid into RNA of brain subcellular fractions of 10-day-old normal and hypothyroid rats. Brain Res., 44, 231–243 (1972)

G19   Gonzalez-Mujica, F. and Mathias, A. P. Studies of nuclei separated by zonal centrifugation from liver of rats treated with thioacetamide. Biochem. J., 132, 163–183 (1973)

G20   Goodman, J. I. and Potter, V. R. The effect of 5-fluorodeoxyuridine on the synthesis of deoxyribonucleic acid pyrimidines in precancerous rat liver. Mol. Pathol. 9, 297–303 (1973)

G21   Gordonoff, T. and Schneeberger, E. W. Orotsäure und Leberzirrhose. Int. Z. Vitaminforsch., 30, 206 (1959)

G22   Gray, D. W. G. and Mowat, A. P. Effects of aspartic acid, orotic acid, and glucose on serum bilirubin concentrations in infants born before term. Arch. Dis. Child., 46, 123–124 (1971)

G23   Grigoryan, L. A. Pyrimidine derivatives. XLIII. Synthesis of some orotic acid analogues. Arm. Khim. Zh., 28, 564–571 (1975) (Russ.)

G24   Gröbner, W. and Kelley, W. N. Effect of allopurinol and its metabolic derivatives on the configuration of human orotate phosphoribosyl-transferase and orotidine 5'-phosphate decarboxylase. Biochem. Pharmacol., 24, 379–384 (1975)

G25 Gröbner, W. and Zöllner, N. Zur Beeinflussung der Purin- und Pyrimidinsynthese durch Allopurinol. Klin. Wochenschr., 53, 255–260 (1975)

G26 Gröbner, W. and Zöllner, N. Störungen des menschlichen Pyrimidinstoffwechsels. Münch. Med. Wochenschr., 37 (Suppl.), 1453–1456 (1975)

G27 Gröbner, W., Meurer, M. and Zöllner, N. Über den Einfluss von Osmadizon auf Serumharnsäure sowie renale Harnsäure-, Oxypurin- und Orotsäureausscheidung Gesunder. Presented at the 82nd Tag. Dtsch. Ges. Inn. Med. (Wiesbaden), April 25–29 (1976)

G28 Gröbner, W. and Zöllner, N. The influence of dietary purines and pyrimidines on purine and pyrimidine biosynthesis in man. Inf. Ther., 4, 305–307 (1977)

G29 Grozdanovic, J., Vich, Z. and Truxova, G. Combined effect of 6-azauridine and irradiation in vivo and in vitro. Stud. Biophys., 10, 133–136 (1968)

G30 Gyorgy, G. Orotic acid in food milk powders. Am. J. Clin. Nutr., 23 (1970)

H

H1 Hadjiolova, K. V., Golovinsky, E. V. and Hadjiolov, A. A. The site of action of 5-fluoroorotic acid on the maturation of mouse liver ribonucleic acids. Biochim. Biophys. Acta, 319, 373–382 (1973)

H2 Händel, A., Hinkel, G. K., Kintzel, H.-W. and Schwarze, R. Untersuchungen über die medikamentöse Beeinflussung des Serumbilirubinspiegels Neugeborener. Paediatr. Paedol., 8, 307–315 (1973)

H3 Hallanger, L. E., Laakso, J. W. and Schultze, M. O. Orotic acid in milk. J. Biol. Chem., 202, 83–89 (1953)

H4 Hamuro, Y. Effect of adrenal and hypophyseal hormones on the development of fatty liver in rats fed orotic acid. Endocrinology, 90, 200–206 (1972)

H5 Handschuhmacher, R. E., Creasey, W. A., Jaffe, J. J., Pasternak, C. A. and Hankin, L. Biochemical and nutritional studies on the induction of fatty livers by dietary orotic acid. Proc. Natl. Acad. Sci. USA, 46, 178–186 (1960)

H6 Hapke, H. J., Sterner, W., Heisler, E. and Brauer, H. Toxicological studies with kavaform. Farmaco Ed. Prat., 26, 692–720 (1971)

H7 Hashimoto, S. Effects of nucleic acid precursors on liver injuries. I. Treatment of liver injury induced by low protein, amino acid imbalanced diet with AICA and AICA orotate in massive doses. J. Vitaminol. 13, 9–18 (1976)

H8 Hashimoto, S. Effects of nucleic acid precursors on liver injuries. II. The influences of AICA and AICA orotate on metabolism in liver injuries and their clinical significances. J. Vitaminol. 13, 19–25 (1967)

H9 Hatchwell, L. C. and Milner, J. A. Amino acid induced aciduria. J. Nutr., 108, 578–584 (1978)

H10 Hatchwell, L. C. and Milner, J. A. Factors affecting amino acid induced orotic aciduria in rats. J. Nutr., 108, 1976–1981 (1978)

H11 Hatfield, P. J., Simmonds, H. A., Cameron, J. S., Jones, A. S. and Cadenhead, A. Effects of allopurinol and oxonic acid on pyrimidine metabolism in the pig. Adv. Exp. Med. Biol., 41, 637–638 (1974)

H12 Hay, R. V., Dubien, L. H. and Getz, G. S. Sialylation in antitrypsin deficiency. N. Engl. J. Med., 292, 1031–1032 (1975)

H13 Hayano, K., Tsubone, T., Azuma, I. and Yamamura, Y. The prevention of the orotic acid fatty liver by the administration of 5-aminoimidazolecarboxamide. J. Biochem., 52, 379–380 (1962)

H14 Hayashi, T. T. and Macfarlane, K. Changes in the incorporation of different RNA precursors into the maternal liver during pregnancy. Nature (London), 246, 94–96 (1973)

H15 Heinrich, H. C. Vitamin-Stoffwechsel und Vitamin-Therapie bei Lebererkrankungen. Unter besonderer Berücksichtigung des Vitamin B$_{12}$, der Folsäure und anderer B-Vitamine. Med. Welt, 35, 1791–1801 (1966)

H16 Heinrich, H. C. Therapeutische Wirksamkeit der B-Vitamine und anderer Medikamente bei chronischem Leberparenchymkrankheiten? Muench. Med. Wochenschr., 110, 2311–2314 (1968)

H17 Heinrich, H. J. Medikamentöse Behandlung chronischer Leberschäden. Ergebnisse mit einer neuen leberwirksamen Substanz. Aerztl. Praxis, 26, 65–67 (1974)

H18 Heitefuss, R. Influence of actinomycin on *Puccinia graminis tritici* on wheat and the incorporation of orotic acid-[^{14}C] and uridine [^{3}H] in host and parasite. Phytopathol. Z., 69, 107–114 (1970) (Germ.)

H19 Helene, C. and Charlier, M. Photosensitized splitting of pyrimidine dimers by indole derivatives. Biochem. Biophys. Res. Commun., 43, 252–257 (1971)

H20 Herbert, M. A. and Johns, H. E. Flash photolysis studies of orotic acid. Photochem. Photobiol., 14, 693–704 (1971)

H21 Herbert, M. A. and Johns, H. E. Flash photolysis. II. Photoreduction of orotic acid in aqueous medium. J. Phys. Chem., 77, 1199–1204 (1973)

H22 Herbst, J. J., Fortin-Magana, R. and Sunshine, P. Relationship of pyrimidine biosynthetic enzymes to cellular proliferation in rat intestine during development. Gastroenterology, 59, 240–246 (1970)

H23 Herrmann, E. C., Dunn, J. H. and Schmidt, R. R. DEAE paper chromatography to separate intermediates of the pyrimidine biosynthetic pathway and to assay aspartate transcarbamylase and dihydroorotase activities. Analyt. Biochem., 53, 478–483 (1973)

H24 Hinkel, G. K., Kemmer, Ch., Kintzel, H. W., Roschlau, G. and Schwarze, R. Zur Frage der Nebenwirkung der Orotsäure bei Frühgeborenen. Kinderaerztl. Prax., 38, 247–252 (1970)

H25 Hinkel, G. K., Kintzel, H.-W. and Schwarze, R. Der

Einfluß von Orotsäure auf den Serumbilirubinspiegel Frühgeborener. Kinderaerztl. Prax., 38, 323–328 (1970)

H26   Hinkel, G. K., Schwarze, R. and Kintzel, H.-W. Der Einfluß einer kombinierten Behandlung mit Orotsäure und Phenobarbital auf den Serumbilirubinspiegl Frühgeborener. Schweiz. Med. Wochenschr., 102, 331–335 (1972)

H27   Hinkel, G. K., Kintzel, H.-W. and Schwarze, R. Untersuchungen über die Prophylaxe der Hyperbilirubinämie Früh- und Neugeborener mit Orotsäure. Dtsch. Gesundheitwes., 27, 2414–2419 (1972)

H28   Hinkel, G. K., Schwarze, R. and Kintzel, H.-W. Optimale Orotsäuredosierung zur Verhütung der toxischen Hyperbilirubinämie Frühgeborener. Acta. Paediatr. Acad. Sci. Hung. 13, 367–375 (1972)

H29   Hinkel, G. K., Kintzel, H.-W., Schwarze, R. and Händel, A. Untersuchungen über die Prophylaxe der Hyperbilirubinämie Neugeborener mit Orotsäure und Enzyminduktoren. Presented at the 5th Gastroenterologen Kongress, September 10–12 (1973), Leipzig

H30   Hinkel, G. K. and Le Petit, G. Untersuchungen über die enterale Resorption der Orotsäure bei Neugeborenen. Paediatr. Grenzgeb., 12, 63–69 (1973)

H31   Hinkel, G. K. and Kemmer, Ch. Elektronenmikroskopische Untersuchungen über Leberveränderungen bei Frühgeborenen nach Enzyminduktion. Paediatr. Grenzgeb., 12, 201–213 (1973)

H32   Hinkel, G. K. and Richter, K. Untersuchungen zur Proteinbindung der Orotsäure. Paediatr. Grenzgeb., 12, 215–221 (1973)

H33   Hirsch, W. and Smerlings, H. Medikamentöse Therapie von Lebererkrankungen mit Hepatofalk. Ther. Ggw., 115, 1719–1754 (1976)

H34   Hoffman, D. H. and Sweeney, M. J. Orotate phosphoribosyl transferase and orotidylic acid decarboxylase activities in liver and Morris hepatomas. Cancer Res., 33, 1109–1112 (1973)

H35   Hogans, A. F., Guroff, G. and Udenfriend, S. Origin of pyrimidines for biosynthesis of neural RNA in the rat. J. Neurochem., 18, 1699–1710 (1971)

H36   Hokanson, J. T., O'Brien, W. R., Idemoto, J. and Schafer, I. A. Carrier detection in ornithine transcarbamylase deficiency. J. Pediatr., 93, 75–78 (1978)

H37   Holtzman, J. L. Effect of orotic acid and adenine sulfate on the levels of aniline hydroxylase and ethylmorphine N-demethylase in male and female rats. Fed. Proc., 26, 462 (1967)

H38   Holtzman, J. L. and Gillette, J. R. Effect of dietary orotic acid and adenine sulfate on hepatic microsomal enzymes in male and female rats. Biochem. Pharmacol., 18, 1927–1933 (1969)

H39   Hoogenraad, N. J. and Lee, D. C. Effect of uridine on de novo pyrimidine biosynthesis in rat hepatoma cells in culture. J. Biol. Chem., 249, 2763–2768 (1974)

H40   Horan, P. K. and Snipes, W. Electron spin resonance of irradiated single crystals of orotic acid. Radiat. Res., 41, 24–38 (1970)

H41   Howell, R. R. Hereditary orotic aciduria. In Zöllner, N. and Gröbner, W. (eds) Handbuch Inn. Med., Fuenfte Aufl. 7, Teil 3, pp. 635–650. (Berlin: Springer) (1976)

H42   Hurlbert, R. B. and Potter, V. R. A survey of the metabolism of orotic acid in the rat. J. Biol. Chem., 195, 257–270 (1952)

H43   Hurlbert, R. and Reichard, P. Conversion of orotic acid to uridine phosphates by soluble enzymes of liver. Acta Chem. Scand., 8, 701 (1954)

I

I1   Ignat'ev, M. V. Therapeutic use of potassium orotate. Kardiologiia, 9, 91–92 (1969) (Russ.)

I2   Irsigler, K., Flegel, U., Kühn, P., Schubert, H., Ivan, E., Biro, L. and Szekely, L. Verbessert Magnesium-Orotat die

Wirkung lipidsenkender Pharmaka? Int. J. Clin. Pharmacol., 8, 85–95 (1973)

I3   Ito, K. and Uchino, H. Control of pyrimidine biosynthesis in human lymphocytes. Induction of glutamine-utilizing carbamyl phosphate synthetase and operation of orotic acid pathway during blastogenesis. J. Biol. Chem., 246, 4060–4065 (1971)

I4   Ivanov, V. R., Ivanova, L. S. and Dubnikova, L. A. Effect of potassium orotate on the activity of certain enzymes in blood serum during pulmonary regeneration. Farmakol. Reparativn. Regeneratsii., 3, 68 (1977). From Ref. Zh. Biol. Khim. (1977) (Russ.) Abstr. No. 23Ch367

I5   Iwata, H., Kobayashi, K., Suga, Y. and Mochizuki, K. Nutritional effects of distiller's residues and orotic acid. Vitamins, 45, 321–326 (1972) (Japan.)

J

J1   Janakidevi, K. and Smith, M. J. H. Effects of salicylate on the incorporation of orotic acid into nucleic acids of mouse tissues in vivo. J. Pharm. Pharmacol., 22, 51–55 (1970)

J2   Janakidevi, K. and Smith, M. J. H. Effects of salicylate on RNA polymerase activity and on the incorporation of orotic acid and thymidine into the nucleic acids of rat foetuses in vitro. J. Pharm Pharmacol., 22, 249–252 (1970)

J3   Janssen, A., Gröbner, W., Zöllner, N. Untersuchungen über den Einfluss verschiedener Purin- und Pyrimidinderivate auf die Pyrimidinsynthese des Menschen. Presented at the 82nd Tag. Dtsch. Ges. Inn. Med. (Wiesbaden), April 25–29 (1976)

J4   Japanese patent. Mikrobiologische Synthese der Orotsäure. Jap. Pat. 7106, 397, (1971) (CA 74, 110409a)

J5   Jasinskas, L. Synthesis and biological studies of some hydrazine derivatives of orotic acid. Sin. Izuch. Fiziol. Aktiv. Veshchestv, Mater. Konf., 105–108 (1971) (CA 79, 78718r)

J6   Joseph, P. K. and Subrahmanyam, K. Renal gluconeogenesis in partially hepatectomized, orotic acid fed and semi-starved rats. Indian J. Biochem., 7, 261–263 (1970)

K

K1   Kaidin, D. A. Effect of orotic acid on the concentration of cholesterol and total lipids in the blood and organs of rabbits with experimental atherosclerosis. Toksikologie, 36, 571–574 (1973)

K2   Kalra, J. and Wheldrake, J. F. Evidence that the stimulation of precursor incorporation into RNA of rat kidney by aldosterone is mainly an effect on uptake. FEBS Lett., 25, 298–300 (1972)

K3   Kaneti, J., Golovinsky, E., Yukhnovsky, I. and Genchev, D. A study of some orotic acid derivatives and analogues by Huckel's method of molecular orbitals. I. A theoretical study of the active site of orotidine-5'-phosphate pyrophosphorylase. J. Theor. Biol., 26, 19–27 (1970)

K4   Kaneti, J. and Golovinsky, E. Quantitative relations between the electronic structure and biological activity of some analogs of orotic acid. Chem. Biol. Interactions, 3, 421–428 (1971)

K5   Karska, B., Tscherning, U., Herve, G. and Fromageot, P. Preparative biosynthesis of [^{14}C] orotic acid. J. Labelled Comp., 7, 553–555 (1971)

K6   Kaufmann, E., Sidransky, N. and Shinozuka, H. Incorporation of [^{14}C] orotic acid into RNA of different sized nucleoli of rat livers following partial hepatectomy or after force-feeding a threonine-devoid diet. Exp. Cell Res., 55, 130–132 (1968)

K7   Kaufmann, R., Helmer, K. H., Kouros, M. and Kuns, W. Influence of halothane and phenobarbital on the incorporation of orotic acid into pyrimidinenucleotides, poly (A)-RNA and ribosomal RNA of liver. Arch. Pharm., 293 (Suppl.), 123 (1976)

K8   Kavipurapu, P. R. and Jones, M. E. Purification, size and properties of the complex of orotate phosphoribosyltransferase:orotidylate decarboxylase from mouse Ehrlich ascites carcinoma. J. Biol. Chem., 251, 5589–5599 (1976)

K9   Keiding, S. Effect of orotate on ethanol and galactose metabolism in perfused rat liver. Digestion, 12, 4–6 (1975)

K10   Keiding, S. and Vinterby, A. Orotate decreases the inhibitory effect of ethanol on galactose elimination in the perfused rat liver. Biochem. J., 160, 715–720 (1976)

K11   Kelley, W. N. and Beardmore, Th. D. Allopurinol: alteration in pyrimidine metabolism in man. Science, 169, 388–390 (1970)

K12   Kelley, W. N., Fox, J. and Wyngaarden, J. B. Regulation of purine biosynthesis in cultured human cells. I. Effects of orotic acid. Biochim. Biophys. Acta, 215, 512–516 (1970)

K13   Kelley, W. N., Greene, M. L., Fox, J. H., Rosenbloom, F. M., Levy, R. I. and Seegmiller, J. E. Effects of orotic acid on purine and lipoprotein metabolism in man. Metab. Clin. Exp., 19, 1025–1035 (1970)

K14   Kennedy, J. Distribution, subcellular localization and product inhibition of dihydroorotate oxidation in the rat. Arch. Biochem. Biophys., 157, 369–373 (1973)

K15   Kennedy, J. Dihydroorotase from rat liver: purification, properties and regulatory role in pyrimidine biosynthesis. Arch. Biochem. Biophys., 160, 358–365 (1974)

K16   Keppler, D., Rudigier, J., Reutter, W., Lesch, R. and Decker, K. Orotate prevents galactosamine hepatitis. Hoppe-Seyler's Z. Physiol. Chem., 351, 102–104 (1970)

K17   Keppler, D., Rudigier, J. and Decker, K. Enzymic determination of uracil nucleotides in tissues. Anal. Biochem., 38, 105–114 (1970)

K18   Keppler, D. and Henning, H. Neues Präparat: Aicorat. Frage und Antwort. Internistische Prax., 686 (1972)

K19   Keppler, D., Pausch, J. and Decker, K. Selective uridine triphosphate deficiency induced by D-galactosamine in liver and reversed by pyrimidine nucleotide precursors. J. Biol. Chem., 249, 211–216 (1974)

K20 Kheinonen, I. and Makeeva, N. The influence of potassium orotate on the course of myocardial infarction. Kardiologija (Moskva), 10, 31–35 (1970)

K21 Kidder, G. W. and Nolan, L. L. Pteridine-requiring dihydroorotate hydroxylase from Crithidia fasciculata. Biochem. Biophys. Res. Commun., 53, 926–936 (1973)

K22 Kieffer, F., Solms, J. and Egli, R. H. Vorkommen von Nucleotiden und verwandten Verbindungen in Milch und Milchprodukten. Z. Lebensm. Unters. Forsch., 125, 346–350 (1964/65)

K23 Kiermeier, F. and Buckl, A. Einflüsse auf den Orotsäuregehalt in Kuhmilch. Z. Lebensm. Unters. Forsch., 138, 284–294 (1968)

K24 Kinet, J. M., Bodson, M., Alvinia, A. M. and Bernier, G. Inhibition of flowering in Sinapis alba after the arrival of the floral stimulus at the meristem. Z. Pflanzenphysiol., 66, 49–63 (1971)

K25 Kinsella, J. E. Protein and lipoperoxide levels in orotic acid induced fatty livers. Can. J. Biochem., 45, 1206–1211 (1967)

K26 Kinsella, J. E. Increased lipoperoxide content of orotic acid-induced fatty liver. Biochim. Biophys. Acta, 137, 205–207 (1967)

K27 Kintanar, Q. L. Mechanisms of the fatty liver and the hypolipidemia induced by orotic acid in the rat. Diss. Abstr. Int. B., 31, 2530 (1970)

K28 Kintzel, H.-W., Hinkel, G. K. and Schwarze, R. The decrease in the serum bilirubin level in premature infants by orotic acid. Acta Paediatr. Scand., 60, 1–5 (1971)

K29 Kintzel, H.-W., Braun, W., Hinkel, G. K., Koslowski, H. and Schwarze, R. The effect of orotic acid on the bilirubin-absorptive power of plasma albumin in newborn infants. Acta Paediatr. Scand., 61, 703–705 (1972)

K30 Kintzel, H.-W., et al. Prophylaxe der toxischen Hyperbilirubinämie. Induktoren-Kombination effektiv/Alle untergewichtigen Neugeborenen behandeln. Prax. Kurier, 48 (1974)

K31 Klain, G. J. The effect of orotic acid and cold stress on lipogenesis in white adipose tissue. Biochim. Biophys. Acta, 144, 174–176 (1967)

K32　Klain, G. J., Sullivan, F. J. and Meikle, A. W. Dietary orotic acid and lipogenesis in the rat. J. Nutr., 100, 1431–1436 (1970)

K33　Kleihues, P. *N*-methyl-*N*-nitrosourea induced changes in the labeling by [^{14}C] orotate of RNA and acid-soluble fractions in rat kidney and liver. Chem. Biol. Interact., 5, 309–315 (1972)

K34　Kleimenova, N. N., Alekseeva, S. P. and Belenky, E. E. Effect of potassium orotate on the ultrastructure of muscle fibers of the heart in experimental myocardial infarction. Byull. Eksp. Biol. Med., 75, 105–109 (1973) (Russ.)

K35　Klosa, J. Synthese eines wasserlölischen Orotsäuresalzes. Artzneim. Forsch., 26, 1532 (1976)

K36　Klubes, P., Fay, P. J. and Cerna, I. Effects of chlorpromazine on cell wall biosynthesis and incorporation of orotic acid into nucleic acids in *Bacillus megaterium*. Biochem. Pharmacol., 20, 265–277 (1971)

K37　Knight, D. M. and Jones, E. E. Regulation of *Escherichia coli* ornithine transcarbamylase by orotate. J. Biol. Chem., 252, 5928–5930 (1977)

K38　Kobayashi, K., Tabe, K., Sasaki, I. and Nakamura, T. Clinical studies of AICA orotate (Alcamin) in chronic hepatic diseases. Asian Med. J., 6, 1089–1096 (1963)

K39　Kobori, S. and Kawakami, S. Polarographic studies on food additives. I. Polarographic reduction wave of orotic acid. Utsunomiya Daigaku Kyoikugakubu Kiyo, Dai 2 bu, 26, 27–35 (1976) (Japan)

K40　Kochakian, C. D. and Hill, J. Effect of castration and androgens on the incorporation of 6-[^{14}C] orotic acid into the prostate and seminal vesicles of the mouse. Steroids, 15, 777–788 (1970)

K41　Kochakian, C. D., Dubovsky, J. and Broulik, P. Effect of nutritive state and precursor dose on the incorporation of orotic acid and uridine into kidney and liver of normal, castrated and androgen-treated mice. Endocrinology, 90, 531–537 (1972)

K42 Köcher, Z., Habermannova, S., Cerhova, M. and Suva, J. The influence of orotic acid on liver parenchyma. IV. Changes in serum and liver lipids due to chronic carbon tetrachloride intoxication. Acta Vitaminol., 6, 269–275 (1964)

K43 Kolla, V. E., Bilich, G. L., Porollo, V. I., Otmakhov, V. N. and Suslova, O. I. Effect of potassium orotate on compensatory hypertrophy of the remaining lung after left-sided pulmonectomy. Eksp. Khir. Anesteziol., 4, 35–38 (1975) (Russ.)

K44 Kolos, G., Williams, J. F. and Hickie, J. B. Biochemical studies in myocardial hypertrophy and metabolic support of the acutely stressed myocardium. Adv. Cardiol., 12, 106–115 (1974)

K45 Koreshkova, N. A., Matveenko, V. N. and Fedorov, N. A. Comparative effectiveness of the biosynthesis of pyrimidine nucleotides by de novo and salvage pathways in a rat bone marrow culture. Mater. Resp. S'ezda Gematol. Transfuziologov Beloruss., (Pub. 1973) 42–45 (Russ.)

K46 Kotaki, A., Okumura, M., Hasan, S. H. and Yagi, K. Myo-inositol. V. Effect of myo-inositol on the prevention of fatty liver induced by orotic acid. J. Vitaminol., 16, 75–79 (1970)

K47 Koudela, K., Sova, Zd., Trefny, D., Hrdinova, A., Vrbenska, A., Nemec, Z., Sevcikova, I. and Kolomaznikova, J. Influence of orotic acid on domestic chickens. Biol. Chem. Vvz. Zvířăt, 10, 29–40 (1974) (Czech.)

K48 Kratzsch, K.-H. and Petzold, H. Der Einfluss von Orotsäure auf die Tetrachlorkohlenstoff-Fibrose des Kaninchens. Ber. Sek. Inn. Med., 4, 284–285 (1966)

K49 Kraushaar-Baldauf, E. and Rotta, L. Die Orotsäure als Wuchsstoff höherer Pflanzen. A.F., 8, 300–301 (1958)

K50 Krauz, V. A. Effect of ethipyrol and orotic acid on the training and memory of dogs. Farmakol. Toksikol. (Moscow), 35, 537–541 (1972) (Russ.)

K51 Kretchmer, N., Hurwitz, R. and Raiha, N. Some aspects of urea and pyrimidine metabolism during development. Biol. Neonat., 9, 187–196 (1965/66)

K52 Kriska, M., Reinis, St. and Suva, J. Influence of orotic acid on the hepatic parenchyma. VIII. Changes of the localization of acid phosphatase and AS-esterase in the liver after application of orotic acid and vitamin B_{12}. Acta Histochem., 23, 80–85 (1966)

K53 Krooth, R. S. Molecular models for pharmacological tolerance and addiction. Ann. N.Y. Acad. Sci., 179, 548–560 (1971)

K54 Krooth, R. S. Regulation of uridine 5'-monophosphate synthesis in human diploid cells. Symp. Int. Soc. Cell Biol., 9, 43–68 (1971)

K55 Krooth, R. S., Pan, Y.-L. and Pinsky, L. Orotidine 5'-monophosphate decarboxylase activity of crude extracts of human cells. Biochem. Genet., 8, 133–148 (1973)

K56 Krooth, R. S., Lam, G. F. M. and Chen Kiang, S. Y. Oxipurinol and orotic aciduria: effect on the orotidine-5'-monophosphate decarboxylase activity of cultured human fibroblasts. Cell, 3, 55–57 (1974)

K57 Krug, M., Ott, T., Schulzeck, K. and Mathies, H. Effects of orotic acid and pirazetam on cortical bioelectrical activity in rabbits. Psychopharmacology (Berlin), 53, 73–78 (1977)

K58 Krukow, N. and Brodersen, R. Toxic effects in the Gunn rat of combined treatment with bilirubin and orotic acid. Acta Paediatr. Scand., 61, 697–703 (1972)

K59 Kruski, A. W. and Narayan, K. A. Effect of orotic acid and cholesterol on the synthesis and composition of chicken (*Gallus domesticus*). Int. J. Biochem., 7, 635–638 (1976)

K60 Kubaček, L., Ondřejicka, M., Mikulecky, M. and Hantak, I. The mathematical model of intermittent drug action. Medinfo, 74, 875–877 (1974)

K61 Kublickiene, O. Effect of orotic acid in guinea pigs poisoned with carbon tetrachloride. Mater. Nauch. Konf. Vses. Obshchest. Gel'mintol. 2, 158–160 (1968) (Russ.)

K62 Kublickiene, O., Svetlaviciene, L. and Cheremnykh, E.

Effect of orotic acid on the course of a pathological process in the liver of sheep after vermifuge treatment during fascioliasis. Probl. Parazitol. Pribaltike, Mater. Nauch.-Koord. Konf. 4th, 117–119 (1968) (Russ.)

K63   Kublickiene, O. Stimulation of the reverse development of changes in the liver of animals poisoned with carbon tetrachloride. Dokl. Nauch. Konf. Anat., Gistol. Embriol. Est., Latv. Litvy 1969, 163–167 (1973) (Russ.)

K64   Kubonoya, J., Kimura, M. and Hongo, A. Clinical effectiveness of 4-amino-5-imidazole carboxamide orotate (Aicamin) on liver disease. Asian Med. J., 7, 196–198 (1964)

K65   Kühn, H. A. Umfrage: leberschutzpräparate. Int. Prax., 3 (Suppl.), 517 (1974)

K66   Kushima, K. Studies on effect of orotic acid in liver damage. Med. J. Osaka Univ., 9, 549–565 (1958)

L

L1   Lafarge, C. and Frayssinet, C. Minor role of the *de novo* pathway in the biosynthesis of RNA during fetal and neoplastic liver development in rats. Biochimie, 54, 471–481 (1972) (French)

L2   Lafille, C., Charbonnier, A., Rousselot, P. and Cachin, M. Acide orotique et régénération hépatique après hépatéctomie partielle chez le rat. R.I.H., 17, 429–448 (1967)

L3   Landgraf, R., Hess, J. and Ermisch, A. Der Einfluss von Vasopressin auf die regionale Aufnahme von [^{3}H]-Orotsäure in Rattenhirn. Acta Biol. Med. Ger., 37, 655–658 (1978)

L4   Larson, B. L. and Hegarty, H. M. Orotic acid and pyrimidine nucleotides of ruminant milks. J. Dairy Sci., 60, 1223–1229 (1977)

L5 Laszlo, B. Stimulierung geschädigter Leberzellen. Medikamentöse Behandlung von Fettleber und chronisch aggressiver Hepatitis. Aerztl. Prax., 29, 1113 (1977)

L6 Lazareva, D. N. and Plechev, V. V. Effect of panangin, orotic acid and potassium orotate on the absorbing capacity of the reticuloendothelium system. In Lotsmanov, Yu. A. (ed.), 63–64. (Ufa) (1973) (Russ.)

L7 Lea, M. A., Bullock, J., Khalil, F. L. and Morris, H. P. Incorporation of precursors and inhibitors of nucleic acid synthesis into hepatomas and liver of the rat. Cancer Res., 34, 3414–3420 (1974)

L8 Lee, I. P. Effects of β-diethylaminoethyl-diphenylpropylacetate (SKF 525-A) on biological membranes. II. SKF 525-A induced effects on the growth and uptake of L-amino acids by E. coli (diploid mutant). Biochem. Pharmacol., 22, 1075–1082 (1973)

L9 Lenaz, G., Sechi, A. M. and Borgatti, A. R. Effects of lysine and orotic acid on the brain lipid composition of lysine-deficient rats. Boll. Soc. Ital. Biol. Sper., 44, 2180–2182 (1968) (Ital.)

L10 Levitan, R. and Havivi, E. Effect of hypophysectomy on amino acid, thymidine and orotic acid incorporation into the mucosa of the small bowel. Can. J. Biochem., 48, 828–830 (1970)

L11 Lewan, L., Petersen, I. and Yngner, T. Incorporation of orotic acid into nucleotides and RNA in mouse organs during 60 minutes. Hoppe-Seyler's Z.Physiol. Chem., 356 425–429 (1975)

L12 Lie, T. S., Nakano, H., Gappa, P., Böhmer, F. and Ebata, H. Einfluss von Cholinorotat auf die Azathioprin-Immunosuppression bei Hundeleber-Allotransplantation. Leber Magen Darm, 7, 361 (1974)

L13 Lindenau, E., Böttcher, M., Bunke, H. and Jung, U. Zur medikamentösen Prophylaxe der Neugeborenen-Hyperbilirubinämie. II. Mitteilung: Tierexperimentelle und klinische Erprobung der Dreierkombination Phenobarbital, Orotsäure und Adeninsulfat. Dtsch. Gesundheitwes., 33, 26–30 (1978)

L14   Lindsay, R. H., Cash, A. G. and Hill, J. B. TSH stimulation of orotic acid conversion to pyrimidine nucleotides and RNA in bovine thyroid. Endocrinology, 84, 534–543 (1969)

L15   Lindsay, R. H., Cash, A. G. and Hill, J. B. Mechanism of action of TSH on pyrimidine nucleotide synthesis. Endocrinology, 89, 492–499 (1971)

L16   Lipkan, G. N. Determination of the acute toxicity of some preparations possessing vitamin activity. Farmakol. Toksikol. (Kiev), 6, 127–131 (1971) (Russ.)

L17   Lipkan, G. N. Toxicity of some vitamin preparations in experiments. Farmakol. Toksikol. (Kiev), 7, 128–131 (1972) (Russ.)

L18   Lipkan, G. M. and Maksyutina, N. P. Use of increased doses of vitamin preparations of B and P groups for the inhibition of experimental inflammatory reactions. Farm. Zh. (Kiev), 28, 59–90 (1973) (Ukrain.)

L19   Lipkan, G. N. and Mokhort, N. A. Antiinflammatory action of several vitamin preparations. Fiziol. Akt. Veschestva, 5, 135–138 (1973) (Russ.)

L20   Loessner, B. and Matthies, H. Effect of intraventricularly administered sodium orotate on a conditional escape reaction in rats. Acta Biol. Med. Ger., 27, 221–224 (1971) (Germ.)

L21   Löw, O., Macnik, G., Arnrich, M. and Urban, J. Studies on Quantitative. I. Correlation between mitoses and binucleated cells during liver regeneration. Z. Mikrosk. Anat. Forsch., 84, 91–100 (1971) (Germ.)

L22   Löw, O., Machnik, G., Arnrich, M., Urban, J., Lemke, H. and Chemnitius, K.-H. Versuche zur medikamentösen Beeinflussung altersbedingter Veränderungen. II. Untersuchungen zur Toxizität von Meklofenoxat-Derivaten. Zentralbl. Pharm., 113 (Suppl.), 693–700 (1974)

L23   Löw, O., Machnik, G., Arnrich, M., Urban, J. and Lemke, H. Versuche zur medikamentösen Beeinflussung altersbedingter Veränderungen. III. Über die Verminderung des Lipofuszingehaltes in den Ganglienzellen des Nucleus reticularis gigantocellularis von Albinoratten nach Orotsäure, Dehydrochlormethyltestosteron und Meklofenoxaorotat. Zentralbl. Pharm., 113 (Suppl.), 701–704 (1974)

L24   Löw, O., Machnik, G., Arnrich, M. and Urban, J. Versuche zur medikamentösen Beeinflussung altersbedingter Veränderungen. IV. Über den Einfluss einer Vorfütterung mit Orotsäure und Dehydrochlormethyltestosteron auf die Leberregeneration nach partieller Hepatektomie. Zentralbl. Pharm., 113 (Suppl.), 705–716 (1974)

L25   Lotz, M., Fallon, H. J. and Smith, L. H. Jr. Excretion of orotic acid and orotidine in heterozygotes of congenital orotic aciduria. Nature (London), 197, 194 (1963)

L26   Lutz, M. P. and Domino, E. F. Some evidence for long term memory retention by orotic acid in rats bar pressing for water. Arch. Int. Pharmacodyn. Ther., 211 (Suppl.), 123–127 (1974)

M

M1   Macleod, P., Mackenzie, S. and Scriver, C. R. Partial ornithine carbamyl transferase deficiency, an inborn error of the urea cycle presenting as orotic aciduria in a male infant. Can. Med. Assoc. J., 107, 405–408 (1972)

M2   Makarenko, L. K. Effect of vitamin B_{15} on cholesterol metabolism during experimental orotic acid-induced fatty liver. In Dauletbakov, M. I. (ed.) Fiziol. Patol. Organov. Pishchevareniya, 96–102 (Karaganda, USSR) (1974) (Russ.)

M3   Makino, K., Kinoshita, T., Satoh, K. and Sasaki, T. Orotic acid as one of the growth-factors of mice. Nature (London), 172, 914–915 (1953)

M4   Mandel, H. G. and Riis, M. Interference of barbiturates with pyrimidine incorporation. II. Structural specificity of the inhibition of orotate uptake in Bacillus cereus. Biochem. Pharmacol., 19, 1867–1877 (1970)

M5   Mandel, H. G., Triester, Sh. R. and Szapary, D. Interference of barbiturates with pyrimidine incorporation. III. Studies on the mechanism of the amobarbital-orotate relationship. Biochem. Pharmacol., 19, 1879–1892 (1970)

M6   Mangoff, S. C. and Milner, J. A. Oxonate-induced hyperuricemia and orotic aciduria in mice. Proc. Soc. Exp. Biol. Med., 157, 110–115 (1978)

M7   Manna, L. and Hauge, S. M. A possible relationship of vitamin B_{12} to orotic acid. J. Biol. Chem., 202, 91 (1953)

M8   Manoilov, S. E. Study of the antiblastic effect of some energy metabolism metabolites. In Astrakhan, V. I. (ed.) 2nd Tezisy Dokl. Vses. Konf. Khimoter. Zlokach. Opukholei, p. 105 (Moscow) (1974) (Russ.)

M9   Marchetti, M., Caldarera, C. M. and Moruzzi, G. Effects of orotic acid and methionine on acid-soluble nucleotides of vitamin B_{12}-deficient chicks. Biochim. Biophys. Acta, 55, 218–220 (1962)

M10   Marchetti, M., Puddu, P. and Caldarera, C. M. Metabolic aspects of "orotic acid fatty liver". Nucleotide control mechanisms of lipid metabolism. Biochem. J., 92, 46–51 (1964)

M11   Marchetti, M. and Puddu, P. Metabolic aspects of "orotic acid fatty liver". Relationship between biotin and fatty liver. Arch. Biochem. Biophys., 108, 468–470 (1964)

M12   Marchetti, M., Viviani, R. and Rabbi, A. Effect of orotic acid on vitamin B_{12}-deficient rats. Nature (London), 178, 805 (1965)

M13   Mardashev, S. R. and Fitsner, A. B. Vliianie nekotorykh barbituratov na biosintez pirimidinov *in vitro*. Vopr. Med. Khim., 13, 303–307, (1967)

M14   Markov, G. G., Dessev, G. N., Russev, G. and Tsanev, R. G. Effect of γ-irradiation on biosynthesis of different types of ribonucleic acids in normal and regenerating rat liver. Biochem. J., 146, 41–45 (1975)

M15   Matsuda, I. and Shirahata, T. Effects of aspartic acid and orotic acid upon serum bilirubin level in newborn infants. Tohoku J. Exp. Med., 90, 133–136 (1966)

M16 Matsushita, S. and Fauburg, B. L. Pyrimidine nucleotide synthesis in the normal and hypertrophying rat heart. Circ. Res., 27, 415–428 (1970)

M17 Matthies, H. and Lietz, W. Der Einfluss von Orotsäure auf das Erlöschen einer bedingten Fluchtreaktion der Ratte. Acta Biol. Med. Ger., 19, 785–787 (1967)

M18 Matthies, H. and Kirschner, M. Die Wirkung von Orotsäure auf den Stabsprungtest der Ratte. Acta Biol. Med. Ger., 19, 789–790 (1967)

M19 Matthies, H. and Lietz, W., Die Bedeutung von Applikationsart und Applikationsdauer für die Wirkung von Orotsäure auf ein einfaches Modell eines Lernvorganges. Acta Biol. Med. Ger., 19, 1053–1057 (1967)

M20 Matthies, H., Fahse, C. and Lietz, W. Effect of RNA-precursors on the maintenance of longterm memory. Psychopharmacologia, 20, 10–15 (1971) (Germ.)

M21 Matthies, H. Intracellular regulation of interneuronal connectivity. Basis of learning and memory processes. Presented at the 3rd Biocybern. Proc. Int. Symp. 1971, 4, 10–17 (1972) (Germ.)

M22 Matthies, H. Pharmacological influence on the teaching and memorization processes. Farmakol. Toksikol. (Moscow), 35, 259–265 (1972) (Russ.)

M23 Matveenko, V. N., Fedorov, N. A., Koreshkova, N. A. and Kurbanova, G. N. Comparative rate of utilization of orotic acid and uridine by human and rat bone marrow cells in a short-term culture. Byull. Eksp. Biol. Med., 74, 99–102 (1972) (Russ.)

M24 Mayfield, E. D., Mossé, H., Burleson, S. S., Lyman, K. and Bresnick, E. Orotic acid-induced alterations in pyrimidine metabolism. Fed. Proc., 26, 292 (1967)

M25 Medical Tribune, Editorial. Orotsäure lebensnotwendig. Med. Tribune, 35 (1970)

M26 Meerson, F. Z., Geinisman, I. U. I. A., Larina, V. N., Rosanova, L. S. and Aleksandrovskaya, M. M. Comparative evaluation of the effects of actinomycin 2703 and of orotic acid on the dimensions of spinal motor neurons subjected to motor load. Dokl. Akad. Nauk. SSSR, 174, 1198–1201 (1967) (Russ.)

M27   Mertz, D. P. and Rusteberg, J. Harnsäurestoffwechsel und Serumkonzentration verschiedener Lipide unter der akuten Wirkung von Orotsäure. MMW., 117, 131–136 (1975)

M28   Mijelic, F. and Jurkovic, N. Amount of orotic acid in milk and cheese. Hrana Ishrana, 15, 299 (1974)

M29   Mikunis, R. I. and Morozova, R. Z. Effect of stimulators of nucleic acid synthesis on the myocardial contractile function in rheumatic heart disease. Kardiologiia, 10, 102–106, (1970) (Russ.)

M30   Miller, B. G. and Baggett, B. Effects of 17 beta-estradiol on the incorporation of pyrimidine nucleotide precursors into nucleotide pools and RNA in the mouse uterus. Endocrinology, 90, 645–656 (1972)

M31   Miller, J. P. Failure of orotic acid to suppress activity of plasma lecithin:cholesterol acyltransferase. Scand. J. Clin. Lab. Invest., 38 138–141 (1978)

M32   Milner, J. and Visek, W. J. Orotic aciduria and arginine deficiency. Nature (London), 245, 211–213 (1973)

M33   Milner, J. A., Wakeling, A. E. and Visek, W. J. Effect of arginine deficiency on growth and intermediary metabolism in rats. J. Nutr., 104, 1681–1689 (1974)

M34   Milner, J. A. and Visek, W. J. Orotate, citrate, and urea excretion in rats fed various levels of arginine. Proc. Soc. Exp. Biol. Med., 147, 754–759 (1974)

M35   Milner, J. A. and Visek, W. J. Urinary metabolites characteristic of urea-cycle amino acid deficiency. Metab. Clin. Exp., 25, 643 (1975)

M36   Milner, J. A., Prior, R. L. and Visek, W. J. Arginine deficiency and orotic aciduria in mammals. Proc. Soc. Exp. Biol. Med., 150, 282–288 (1975)

M37   Milner, J. A. and Visek, W. J. Orotic aciduria in the female rat and its relation to dietary arginine. J. Nutr., 108, 1281–1288 (1978)

M38   Milstein, H. G., Cornell, R. C. and Stoughton, R. B. Urine orotic acid-orotidine levels in azaribine-treated patients with psoriasis. J. Invest. Dermatol., 61, 183–187 (1973)

M39   Mitchell, A. D. and Hoogenraad, N. J. *De novo* pyrimidine nucleotide biosynthesis in synchronized rat hepatoma (HTC) cells and mouse embryo fibroblast (3T3) cells. Exp. Cell Res., 93, 105–110 (1975)

M40   Mitova, M. and Bednařik, B. Influencing heart necroses caused by application of isoproterenol, potassium orotate. Scr. Med. Fac. Med. Univ. Brun. Purkynianae, 49, 259–263 (1976)

M41   Miyamoto, M. Der Einbau von [^{14}C] Orotat in die DNA und RNA. Biochim. Biophys. Acta, 272, 612–622 (1972)

M42   Monserrat, A. J., Porta, E. A. and Hartcroft, W. St. Orotic acid effects on the kidney. Changes in choline-deficient weanling rats. Arch. Pathol., 87, 154–163 (1969)

M43   Mori, M. and Tatibana, M. Purification of homogeneous glutamine-dependent carbamyl phosphate synthetase from ascites hepatoma cells as a complex with aspartate transcarbamylase and dihydrorotase. J. Biochem., 78, 239–242 (1975)

M44   Mori, R., Bianco, A. and Cagossi, M. Alterata tolleranza glicidica in corso di cirrosi epatica: Modificazioni endotte dal trattamento con UDPG e Glutatione Ridotto. Fegato, 20, 203–214 (1974)

M45   Moruzzi, G., Rabbi, A., Viviani, R. and Marchetti, M. Ricerche sul contenuto in acido orotico della caseina priva de F.P.A. Acta Vitaminol. 18, 135 (1954)

M46   Moruzzi, G., Marchetti, M., Viviani, R. and Rabbi, A. Acido orotico e fattori proteici animali della caseina. Int. Z. Vitaminforsch., 26, 328–338 (1956)

M47   Moruzzi, G., Viviani, R., Marchetti, M. and Sanguietti, F. Effects of orotic acid on coenzyme A and pantothenic acid of liver in vitamin B_{12} deficiency. Nature (London), 181, 416 (1958)

M48   Motz, R. J. Assay of nonfat milk solids by the determination of orotic acid in milk chocolate and in the milk. Analyst 97, 866–871 (1972)

M49   Moulé, Y. Effects of aflatoxin B1 on the formation of subribosomal particles in rat liver. Cancer Res., 33, 514–520 (1973)

M50   Mowat, A. Double-blind trial of effects of aspartic acid, orotic acid and glucose on serum bilirubin concentrations in infants born before term. Arch. Dis. Child., 46, 397 (1971)

M51   Müller, J. H. Memorandum über Orotsäure in der Geriatrie. (Hamburg: J. H. Müller)

M52   Muenchberg, F., Tsompanidou, G. and Leskova, R. Studies on the presence of orotic acid in milk. Milchwissenschaft, 26, 210–214 (1971) (Germ.)

M53   Murphey, W. H., Patchen, L. and Guthrie, R. Screening tests for argininosuccinic aciduria, orotic aciduria and other inherited enzyme deficiencies using dried blood specimens. Biochem. Genet., 6, 51–59 (1972)

M54   Musil, F., Suva, J. and Prochazkova, B. Le métabolisme des lipides des rats, influences par l'acide orotique, des facteurs lipotropiques, des substances avec le noyau des purines et par le régime purifié. R.I.H., 16, 1269–1274 (1966)

N

N1   Najman, L., Toulova, M. and Herzig, I. Use of orotic acid in chick feeding. Biol. Chem. Vyz. Zviřat., 8, 141–146 (1972) (Czech.)

N2   Nakarai, K., Sasaki, T. and Honda, T. Influence of diet on serum amino acid concentrations in alimentary fatty liver in rats. Presented at the 11th International Congress of Nutrition, August 27–September 1 (1978), Rio de Janeiro

N3   Nassi, P., Cappugi, G., Niccoli, A. and Ramponi, G. Inhibition of horse liver acyl phosphatase by orotic acid. Physiol. Chem. Phys., 5, 109–115 (1973)

N4   Negishi, I. and Aizawa, Y. Effect of orotic acid on the distribution of phosphatidylcholine [^{32}P]. Jpn. J. Pharmacol., 25, 345–348 (1975)

N5 Negret, J. P. Clinical experimentation with Aicamine in hepatic insufficiency. Bordeaux Med., 5, 973–976 (1972) (French)

N6 Nemesansky, E. and Szelenyi, L. Die Wirkung von Magnesium-Orotat und Orotsäure auf die Aktivität lysosomaler Enzyme der Leber. Arzneim. Forsch., 21, 785–787 (1971)

N7 Nemesansky, E., Pavlik, G. and Szelenyi, I. Experimentelle Untersuchungen zur Beeinflussung der Hämodynamik der Arteria coronaria und der Arteria femoralis durch Magnesium-Orotat-Glycinat. Arzneim. Forsch., 21, 791–794 (1971)

N8 Newton, N. A., Cox, G. B. and Gibson, F. The function of menaquinone (vitamin K_2) in *Escherichia coli* K-12. Biochim. Biophys. Acta, 244, 155–166 (1971)

N9 Ng, S. K., Rogers, J. and Sanwal, B. D. Alterations in differentiation and pyrimidine pathway enzymes in 5-azacytidine resistant variants of a myoblast line. J. Cell. Physiol., 90, 361–374 (1977)

N10 Nieper, H. A. The anti-inflammatory and immune-inhibiting effects of calcium orotate on bradythrophic tissues. Agressologie, 10, 349–357 (1969)

N11 Nieper, H. A. Calcium and phosphate metabolism in patients treated with calcium orotate. Agressologie, 12, 401–408 (1971) (French)

N12 Nieper, H. A. Bilanzuntersuchung des Calcium- und Phosphatstoffwechsels an Patienten, die mit Calcium-Orotat behandelt werden. Geriatrie, 9, 184–191 (1972)

N13 Nieper, H. A. Klinische Wirkung von Calcium-diorotat auf Knorpelgewebe. Specifische Funktion in Abhängigkeit vom Pentosen-Stoff wechsel bradytropher Gewebe? Geriatrie, 4 82–86 (1973)

N14 Nieper, H. A. The effects of zinc-orotate. Z. Praeklin. Geriatr., 6, 127–131 (1974)

N15 Nieper, H. A. Clinical treatment with lithium-orotate. Z. Praeklin. Geriatr., 8, 184–186 (1974)

N16 Nieper, H. A. Magnesium-orotate, EPL-substances and clofibrate. Z. Praeklin. Geriatr., 9, 200–203 (1974)

N17   Nieper, H. A. Liver orotate—curative effect of combination of calcium-orotate and lithium-orotate on primary and secondary chronic aggressive hepatitis and liver cirrhosis. Paper presented at the International Academy of Preventive Medicine Symposium, March 9 (1974), Washington.

N18   Nievel, J. G. Transport and incorporation of labelled orotate into ribonucleic acid isolated rat liver perfused with actinomycin D. Biochem. Soc. Trans., 3, 1239–1241 (1975)

N19   Nikolaeva, L. F., Cherpachenko, N. M., Veselova, S. A. and Sokolova, R. I. Mechanisms of drug action on recovery processes of cardiac muscle in myocardial infarction. Circ. Res. Suppl., 3, 202–214 (1974)

N20   Nishigaki, A. Effects of orotic acid and adenine on regenerating rat liver. Wakayama Igaku, 16, 207–213 (1965) (Japan.)

N21   Nissen, K. Zur Therapie der akuten Hepatitis epidemica und der Hepatose. Landarzt Heft, 9, 337–342 (1961)

N22   Nordgren, H. and Stenran, U. Decreased half-life of the RNA of free and membrane-bound ribosomes in the liver of protein-deprived rats. Hoppe-Seyler's Z. Physiol. Chem., 353, 1832–1836 (1972)

N23   Novikoff, P. M., Roheim, P. S., Novikoff, A. B. and Edelstein, D. Production and prevention of fatty liver in rats fed clofibrate and orotic acid diets containing sucrose. Lab. Invest., 30, 732 (1974)

N24   Novikoff, P. M. Experimental fatty liver. I. Production and prevention of fatty liver in rats fed clofibrate and orotic acid diets. II. Reversal of orotic acid induced fatty liver by clofibrate feeding. Diss. Abstr. Int. B., 37, 4279 (1977)

N25   Novikoff, P. M. and Edelstein, D. Reversal of orotic acid-induced fatty liver in rats by clofibrate. Lab. Invest., 36, 215–231 (1977)

N26   Nowack, G. Die Beeinflussung der Blutfette beim generalisierten Sanarelli-Shwartzman-Phänomen durch Nikotinsäure, Orotsäure und kleine Heparindosen. Dissertation, Universität Giessen.

N27 Nussdorfer, G. G. and Mazzocchi, G. Effect of corticosterone on the incorporation of tritiated orotate into adrenocortical cells of hypophysectomized ACTH-treated rats. Experientia, 26, 1374–1375 (1970)

O

O1 Ohlen, J. Neue Gesichtspunkte in der Hepatologie. Prax. Kurier, 49, 6 (1977)

O2 Ohnuma, T., Roboz, J., Shapiro, M. L. and Holland, J. F. Pharmacological and biochemical effects of pyrazofurin in humans. Cancer Res., 37, 2043–2049 (1977)

O3 Okabe, K., Tanaka, T., Fujisawa, K. and Takahashi, T. Metabolic disturbance of nucleotides in damaged liver. Gastroenterol. Japn., 1, 1–10 (1966)

O4 Okonkwo, P. O. and Kinsella, J. E. Orotic acid in food milk powders. Am. J. Clin. Nutr., 22, 532–534 (1969)

O5 Okonkwo, P. O. and Kinsella, J. E. Fatty liver induction by orotic acid contained in skim milk powder. Experientia, 30 993–994 (1974)

O6 Okui, K. and Mtzoguchi, M. Pyrimidine derivatives. VI. Studies on the synthesis of orotic acid, uracil and pyrimido (5,4-D) pyrimidine derivatives. J. Pharm. Soc. Jap., 92, 785–795 (1972) (Jap.)

O7 Ondřejicka, M., Hantak, I., Mikulecky, M. and Kratochvilova, H. Zur Frage der Purinortherapie bei den Leberkrankheiten. Presented at the 5th Gastroenterologen Kongress, September 10–12 (1973) Leipzig.

O8 Ondřejicka, M., Mikulecky, M., Kubaček, L., Hantak, I. and Kratochvilova, H. Probabilistic-statistical model for behaviour of some protein parameters after purines and orotic acid administration in liver diseases. Presented at the Liver Meeting, October (1974) Acapulco, Mexico.

O9 Ondřejicka, M., Mikulecky, M., Hantak, I. and Kratochvilova, H. Die Veränderungen des Laborbildes der chronischen Leberkrankheiten im Verlaufe der intermittierenden Purinotherapie. Bratisl. Lek. Listy, 61, 413–427 (1974)

O10   Ord, M. G. and Stocken, L. A. Uptake of amino acids and nucleic acid precursors by regenerating rat liver. Biochem. J., 129, 175–181 (1972)

O11   Ord, M. G. and Stocken, L. A. Nucleic acid precursor uptake into normal and regenerating rat liver. Biochem. J., 130, 9P (1972)

O12   Ord, M. G. and Stocken, L. A. Uptake of orotate and thymidine by normal and regenerating rat livers. Biochem. J., 132, 47–54 (1973)

O13   Ord, M. G. and Stocken, L. A. Immediate effects of partial hepatectomy on thymidine transport into the liver. In Experimental Liver Injury and Liver Regeneration R. Lesch and W. Reutter (eds) pp. 152–155 (Sratton Medical, New York)

O14   O'Sullivan, W. J. Orotic acid. Aust. N.Z. J. Med., 3, 417–422 (1973)

O15   Ott, T. and Matthies, H. Influence of orotic acid on the significative change of a conditional stimulus. Acta Biol. Med. Ger., 25, 181–183 (1970) (Germ.)

O16   Ott, T. and Matthies, H. Influence of orotic acid and pentetrazole on acquisition and extinction in the model of optic discrimination. Acta Biol. Med. Ger., 26, 79–85 (1971) (Germ.)

O17   Ott, T. and Matthies, H. Influence of orotic acid on the retrograde amnesia caused by electoconvulsive shock. Psychopharmacologia, 20, 16–21 (1971) (Germ.)

O18   Ott, T. and Matthies, H. Influence of 6-azauridine on facilitation of relearning by precursors of ribonucleic acid. Psychopharmacologia, 23, 272–278 (1972) (Germ.)

O19   Ott, T. and Matthies, H. Effects of RNA precursors on development and maintenance of long-term memory. Hippocampal and cortical pre- and post-training application of RNA precursors. Psychopharmacologia, 28, 195–204 (1973)

O20   Ove, P., Adams, R. L. P., Abrams, R. and Lieberman, I. Liver uridine triphosphate after partial hepatectomy. Biochim. Biophys. Acta, 123, 419–421 (1966)

O21 Ozaki, M., Tagawa, S. and Kimura, T. Fermentation products of *Streptomyces*. I. Accumulation of orotic acid and orotidine by a mutant of *Streptomyces showdoensis*. Hakka To Taisha, 26, 24–30 (1972) (Japan.)

O22 Ozaki, M. and Kimura, T. Fermentation products of *Streptomyces*. II. Mechanism of the accumulation of orotic acid and orotidine by a mutant of *Streptomyces showdoensis*. Hakko To Taisha, 26, 31–33 (1972) (Japan.)

P

P1 Pancheva-Golovinskaya, S., Manolova, N. and Golovinskii, E. The effect of various analogs and derivatives of orotic acid on plaque formation by pseudorabies virus. Vopr. Virusol., 15, 354–356 (1970) (Russ.)

P2 Paroli, E., Samueli, F. and Valeri, P. Interazione della benzilpenicillina con la eliminazione biliare della bilirubina e della bromosulfoftaleina: effetto di alcune frazioni epatiche e di loro costituenti. Fegato, 19, 293–300 (1973)

P3 Pasquali, P., Landi, L., Caldarera, C. M. and Marchetti, M. Effects of orotic acid on dihydrofolate dehydrogenase and on tetrahydrofolate-dependent enzymes in the chick liver. Biochim. Biophys. Acta, 158, 482–484 (1968)

P4 Pates, M. M. and Buyanovskaya, O. A. Influence of orotic acid on the phagocytic activity of leukocytes. Bjull. Eksp. Biol. Med., 63, 76 (1967) (Russ.)

P5 Pates, M. M. and Buyanovskaya, O. A. The effect of orotic acid on erythrocyte and granulocyte development in the bone marrow. Bjull. Eksp. Biol. Med., 64, 27–29 (1967) (Russ.)

P6 Pates, M. M., Tseitina, A. I., Pomerantseva, I. I., Tunitskaya, T. A., Kurkina, V. S. and Turetskaya, I. M. Zashchitnoe deistvie orotovoi kisloty na pechen pri vozdeistvii toksicheskikh veshchestv v malykh dozakh. Farmakol. Toksikol., 31, 717–719 (1968)

P7   Pates, M. M., Belenky, E. E. and Buyanovskaya, O. A. The mechanism of the stimulating effect of orotic acid on the phagocytic activity of leukocytes. Bjull. Eksp. Biol. Med., 68, 85–86 (1969) (Russ.)

P8   Pates, M. M., Buyanovskaya, O. A., Kurkina, V. S., Pavlov, G. T., Pomerantseva, I. I., Tunitskaya, T. A., Turetskaya, I. M. and Tseitina, A. I. A. Effect of vitamin B_{12} and folic acid on protective effect of orotic acid. Farmakol. Toksikol., 32, 604–607 (1969) (Russ.)

P9   Pates, M. M., Buyanovskaya, O. A. and Tunitskaya, T. A. Effect of orotic acid on hemopoiesis during its administration with vitamin B_{12} and folic acid. Farmakol. Toksikol., 32, 729–731 (1969) (Russ.)

P10   Pates, M. M., Belenky, E. E., Pavlov, G. T., Kurkina, V. S., Tunitskaya, T. A. and Turetskaya, I. M. Effect of orotic acid on hemopoiesis following the administration of thiophosphamide. Farmakol. Toksikol. 33, 355–357 (1970) (Russ.)

P11   Pates, M. M. Antitoxic properties of orotic acid. K. Mekh. Deistviya Vitam. Zhivotn. Rast. Organizmy, pp. 18–25 (1971) (Russ.)

P12   Pates, M. M. Effect of orotic acid lysozyme activity of the blood serum. Novoe Biokhim. Fiziol. Vitamin. Ferment, pp. 9–16 (1972) (CA 79 (1973) 51711w) (Russ.)

P13   Pausch, J., Keppler, D. and Decker, K. Activity and distribution of the enzymes of uridylate synthesis from orotate in animal tissues. Biochim. Biophys. Acta, 258, 395–403 (1972)

P14   Pausch, J., Keppler, D. and Decker, K. Increased activities of hepatic orotidine 5'-phosphate pyrophosphorylase and orotidine 5'-phosphate decarboxylase induced by orotate. FEBS Lett. 20, 330–332 (1972)

P15   Pausch, J. and Decker, K. Pyrimidine biosynthesis in liver: studies on feedback control and adaption of enzyme levels. Digestion, 8, 138 (1973)

P16   Petzold, H., Storch, H. and Hohlfeld, R. Der Einfluss von Cholinorotat auf die experimentelle Fettleber der Ratte. Z. Inn. Med., 25, 697–700 (1970)

P17   Petzold, H. and Neupert, A. Enzymhistochemische Befunde an der Rattenleber nach Galaktosaminschädigung und Cholinorotat. Z. Inn. Med., 27, 1087–1090 (1972)

P18   Petzold, H. Hepatic tissue enzymes of the rat with galactosamine hepatitis during the concurrent administration of cholinorotate. Cesk. Gastroenterol. Vyz., 27, 290–292 (1973)

P19   Petzold, H. Enzymhistochemische Untersuchungen an Leberpunktaten und ihre Bedeutung für Diagnose und Prognose von Lebererkrankungen. Aus der Gastroenterologischen Abteilung (Leiter: Professor Dr. H. Petzold) der Medizinischen Klinik der Karl Marx-Universität, Leipzig (Direktor: Professor Dr. R. Emmrich)

P20   Pfeifer, G. D., Michaelis, O. E. and Szepesi, B. Incorporation of radioactive orotic acid and 8-azaguanine into rat liver RNA. Res. Comm. Chem. Pathol. Pharmacol., 9, 779 (1974)

P21   Pfeifer, G. D. and Szepesi, B. Changes in hepatic RNA synthesis in the starve-refeed response of the rat. J. Nutr., 104 (Suppl.), 1178–1184 (1974)

P22   Pharmazell. Orotsäurederivate mit verbesserter Wasserlöslichkeit. PHZ 1971/2 (124) (Patentanmeldung)

P23   Pharmazell. Antiinflammatory L-histidine orotate. R.A.M.P. Fr. Demande 2, 175, 559 (C.A. 80 (1974) 124778f)

P24   Pharmazell. Recovery of heart attack victims. Chem. Eng. News, 52, 14 (1974)

P25   Pickering, R. W., James, G. W. L. and Parker, F. L. Inhibition, by drugs, of galactosamine induced hepatitis in the rat. Arzneim. Forsch., 25, 1591–1592 (1975)

P26   Pidemskii, E. L., Martyusheva, S. M. and Sapko, V. Ya. Effect of potassium orotate on the bile-secreting function of the liver in normal conditions and in experimental hepatitis. Patol. Fiziol. Eksp. Ter., 15, 81–82 (1971) (Russ.)

P27   Pinelli, A. and Colombo, A. Nonsteatotic hypolipemic effect of dimethylaminoethanol orotate in the rat. Riv. Farmacol. Ter., 4, 363–367 (1973)

P28   Platt, D. and Rebscher, H. Der Einfluss von Orotat auf die

Galaktosamin-Hepatitis in Abhängigkeit vom Alter der Tiere. Acta Gerontol., 2, 237–242 (1972)

P29   Platt, D., Leinweber, B. and Rebscher, R. Lichtmikroskopische Veränderungen der Galaktosamin-geschädigten Rattenleber und ihre Beeinflussung durch Orotat—in Abhängigkeit vom Alter der Tiere. Z. Gerontol., 6, 125–130 (1973)

P30   Platt, D. and Rebscher, R. Einfluss von Alter und Orotat auf die Galaktosaminschädigung der Rattenleber. Acta Gerontol., 3, 131–141 (1973)

P31   Pogosova, A. V. and Belenky, E. E. Orotic acid and purine effect on protein biosynthesis in compensatory hyperfunction and hypertrophy of the heart. Vopr. Med. Khim. 15, 343–346 (1969) (Russ.)

P32   Popov, N., Schulzeck, S., Schmidt, S., Pohle, W. and Matthies, H. Incorporation of [^{3}H] orotic acid into RNA from different rat brain regions. Acta Biol. Med. Ger., 26, 469–474 (1971) (Germ.)

P33   Popov, N., Schmidt, S., Schulzeck, S. and Matthies, H. Incorporation of intraventricularly administered (3H)-uridine monophosphate, [^{3}H] cytidine monophosphate, and (14C)-orotic acid into brain and liver RNA of the rat. Acta Biol. Med. Ger., 28, 13–20 (1972) (Germ.)

P34   Porta, E. A., Manning, C. and Hartroft, N. St. The lipotropic action of orotic acid. Arch. Pathol. 86, 217–229, (1968)

P35   Pottenger, L. A. and Getz, G. S. Serum lipoprotein accumulation in the livers of orotic acid-fed rats. J. Lipid Res., 12, 450–459 (1971)

P36   Pottenger, L. A., Frazier, L. E., Dubien, L. H., Getz, G. S. and Wissler, R. W. Carbohydrate composition of lipoprotein apoproteins isolated from rat plasma and from the livers of rats fed orotic acid. Biochem. Biophys. Res. Commun. 54, 770–776 (1973)

P37   Prior, R. L. and Visek, W. J. Effects of urea in rats deprived of arginine. J. Nutr., 103, 1107–1111 (1973)

P38   Prior, R. L., Milner, J. A. and Visek, W. J. Urea, citrate and orotate excretions in growing rats fed amino acid-deficient diets. J. Nutr., 105, 141–146 (1975)

P39   Prior, R. L., Zimber, A. and Visek, W. J. Citric, orotic and other organic acids in rats injected with active or inactive urease. Am. J. Physiol., 228, 828–833 (1975)

P40   Prokop, L. Studies of the vegetative action mechanism of kavain and magnesium orotate. HNO, 18, 399–401 (1970) (Germ.)

P41   Prokop, L. Studies of the vegetative action mechanism of kavain and magnesium orotate. Wien. Med. Wochenschr., 121, 399–402 (1971) (Germ.)

R

R1   Rajalakshmi, S., Sarma, D. S. R. and Sarma, P. S. Studies on orotic acid fatty liver. Biochem. J., 80, 375–378 (1961)

R2   Rajalakshmi, S. and Handschuhmacher, R. E. Control of purine biosynthesis *de novo* by orotic acid *in vivo* and *in vitro*. Biochim. Biophys. Acta, 155, 317–325 (1968)

R3   Rajalakshmi, S., Adams, W. R. and Handschuhmacher, R. E. Isolation and characterization of low density structures from orotic acid-induced fatty livers. J. Cell Biol., 41, 625–636 (1969)

R4   Rajamini, S. and Subrahmanyam, K. Metabolism in orotic acid and thiouracil fed rats. Indian J. Biochem. Biophys., 8, 174–175 (1971)

R5   Rampazzo, F. Controlled clinical trial of arginine-malate associated with cytidine and uridine in secondary liver diseases. Minerva Med., 65, 838 (1974)

R6   Raskin, I. M. Vitamin-like substances. Orotic acid. Vitamins, 470, 81 (1974)

R7   Rauch-Janssen, A., Gröbner, W. and Zöllner, N. Studies on the effect of various purine and pyrimidine derivatives on pyrimidine synthesis in humans. Verh. Dtsch. Ges. Inn. Med., 82, 902 (1976)

R8   Razumova, I. L. and Alekseeva, N. N. Effect of yeast RNA and orotic acid on the regeneration of sectioned nerve fibers. Patol. Fiziol. Eksp. Ter., 17, 76–78 (1973) (Russ.)

R9   Reichard, P. The function of orotic acid in the biogenesis of pyrimidines in slices from regenerating liver. J. Biol. Chem., 197, 391–398 (1952)

R10   Rick, J. T., Oliver, G. W. and Kerkut, G. A. Acquisition. extinction and reacquisition of a conditioned response in the cockroach and the effects of orotic acid. Q. J. Exp. Psychol., 24, 282–286 (1972)

R11   Riede, U. N., Strässle, H., Bianchi, L. and Rohr, H. P. Ultrastructural morphometric analysis of rat liver cell after orotic administration. Exp. Mol. Pathol., 15, 271–280 (1971)

R12   Riede, U., Berli, Th. and Mihatsch, M. Beeinflussung der enchondralen Ossifikation durch exogen verabreichte Orotsäure. Beitr. Pathol. 149, 13–22 (1973)

R13   Riemann, D. Kavaform bei chronischen Innenohrstörungen. Fortschr. Med., 32, 1317 (1970)

R14   Ritter, W. The quantative determination of orotic acid as a possibility for determining milk constituents in foods. Mitt. Geb. Lebensmittelunters. Hyg., 68, 240–250 (1977) (Germ.)

R15   Robinson, J. L. and Larson, B. L. Nucleotide inhibition of postorotate pyrimidine synthesis pathway enzymes of bovine mammary tissue. J. Dairy Sci., 57, 1410–1413 (1974)

R16   Robinson, N., Nievel, J. G. and Anderson, J. Changes in nucleotide metabolism of the liver and fate of (14C) orotate among various pyrimidines at the outset and during induction of drug-metabolizing enzymes and hepatomegaly. Biochem. Soc. Trans., 4, 509–510 (1976)

R17   Rössing, P., Eberhard, H. and Brandenburg, W. Zur Therapie der chronischen Hepatitis und Leberzirrhose mit Purinen und Orotsäure. Dtsch. Med. J., 7, 201–204 (1956)

R18   Rogers, L. E. and Nicolaisen, K. Enzymatic spectrophotometric assay for dihydroorotic acid in serum and urine. Experientia, 28, 1258–1259 (1972)

R19   Roheim, P. S., Switzer, S., Girard, A. and Eder, A. The mechanism of inhibition of lipoprotein synthesis by orotic acid. Biochem. Biophys. Res. Commun. 20, 416–421 (1965)

R20   Roheim, P. S., Switzer, S., Girard, A. and Eder, H. A. Alterations of lipoprotein metabolism in orotic acid-induced fatty liver. Lab. Invest., 15, 21–26 (1966)

R21   Rommel, K., Georg, D., Mähr, G. and Török, M. Wirkungen und Nebenwirkungen der Orotsäure. Med. Welt, 17, 1220–1223 (1966)

R22   Rommel, K. In Sachen Orotsäure. Prax. Kurier, 6 (1967)

R23   Rommel, K. and Georg, D. Orotsäure–Nebenwirkungen? Med. Welt, 18, 350 (1967)

R24   Rona, L., Doczy, P. and Marros, T. Behandlung chronischer Leberkrankheiten mit Purin- und Pyrimidinbasen. Aerztl. Prax., 39 (1970)

R25   Ross, J. S., Malamud, D., Caulfield, J. B. and Malt, R. A. Differential labeling with orotic acid and uridine in compensatory renal hypertrophy. Am. J. Physiol. 229, 952–954 (1975)

R26   Rundles, R. W. and Brewer, Sp. S. Jr. Haematologic responses in pernicious anemia to orotic acid. Blood, 13, 99–115 (1958)

R27   Russo, G. and Bonanno, V. Il trattamento con acido orotico in alcuni stati distrofici della prima infanzia. Acta Vitaminol., 15, 61–69 (1961)

S

S1   Sabesin, S. M., Frase, S., Ragland, J. B. and Kuiken, L. Accumulation of lipoproteins in hepatic golgi during induction of fatty liver by orotic acid (OA) feeding. Dig. Dis. Week, May 1976, Miami Beach, Florida

S2   Sabesin, S. M., Frase, S. and Ragland, J. B. Accumulation of nascent lipoproteins in rat hepatic golgi during induction of fatty liver by orotic acid. Lab. Invest., 37, 127–135 (1977)

S3   Sabesin, S. M. and Frase, S. Selective modulation of rat hepatocyte golgi function by induction and reversal of the orotic acid-induced fatty liver. J. Cell Biol. 75, 538 (1977) (1977)

S4   Sabesin, S. M. and Kinnard, M. S. Protective effects of nutritional status on drug-induced fatty liver and hepato-cellular necrosis. Gastroenterology, 72 (1977)

S5   Sabesin, S. M. Ultrastructural features of the mobilization and secretion of very low density lipoproteins (VLDL) following reversal or orotic acid-induced fatty liver in the rat. Gastroenterology, 72 (1977)

S6   Sansotta, S., Celata, G. and Giorgi, C. L'acido orotico quale fattore di accrescimento nell'immaturo. Aggiorn. Pediatr., 11, 363–370 (1960)

S7   Saputo, V. and Nicolis, F. B. Communicazione sul tema di relazione 'Acido orotico: aspetti fisiopatologici sperimentali e clinici'. Acta Vitaminol., 12, 328 (1958)

S8   Sargent, D. R. and Skinner, Ch. G. Thiolesters of orotic acid. J. Med. Chem., 15, 1196 (1972)

S9   Sarma, D. S. R. and Sidransky, H. Studies on orotic acid fatty liver: influence of uridine monophosphate (UMP) on fatty acid synthesis. Fed. Proc., 26, 624 (1967)

S10   Sarma, D. S. R. and Sidransky, H. Biotin deficiency and orotic acid fatty liver in the rat. J. Nutr., 92, 374–376 (1967)

S11   Sarma, D. S. R. and Sidransky, H. Studies on orotic acid fatty liver in rats: factors influencing the induction of fatty liver. J. Nutr., 98, 33–40 (1969)

S12   Sarma, D. S. R., Reid, I. M., Verney, E. and Sidransky, H. Studies on the nature of attachment of ribosomes to membranes in liver. I. Influence of ethionine, sparsomycin, CCl_4, and puromycin on membrane-bound polyribosomal dis-aggregation and on detachment of membrane-bound ribosomes from membranes. Lab. Invest., 27, 39–46 (1972)

S13   Sassoon, H. F., Dror, Y., Watson, J. J. and Johnson, B. S. Dietary regulation of liver glucose-6-phosphate dehydrogenase in the rat: starvation and dietary carbohydrate induction. J. Nutr., 103, 321–335 (1973)

S14   Sauermann, G. Nuclear columns: release of ribonucleopro-
        teins from rat liver nuclei. Biochem. Biophys. Res. Com-
        mun., 56, 155–160 (1974)

S15   Sechi, A. M., Borgatti, A. R. and Lenaz, G. Variation in
        blood and liver cholesterol levels in lysine-deficient rats;
        effects of lysine and orotic acid. Boll. Soc. Ital. Biol. Sper.,
        44, 2183–2185 (1968) (Ital.)

S16   Seifert, J. and Vacha, J. Inhibition of 6-[^{14}C] orotic acid
        incorporation into the cytosine moiety of the ribonucleic
        acid of rat liver cytoplasmic ribosomes after phenobarbital
        administration. Mol. Pharmacol., 9, 259–265 (1973)

S17   Seifert, J. and Vacha, J. Differences in the turnover of
        uridylic and cytidylic acids of rat liver cytoplasmic ribo-
        somes. Arch. Biochem. Biophys., 160, 285–288 (1974)

S18   Seifert, J. and Vacha, J. Cytidine nucleotide biosynthesis
        and the level of cytochrome P-450 in rat liver microsomes
        after administration of colchicine. Arch. Biochem. Bio-
        phys., 172, 106–109 (1976)

S19   Seifert, J. and Vacha, J. Decreased utilization of 2-[^{14}C]
        orotic acid for the synthesis of cytidine nucleotides in rat
        liver after administration of α-hexychlorocyclohexane. Tox-
        icology, 7, 155–161 (1977)

S20   Serra, U., Sacchetti, G. and Della Marca, A. Valutazione in
        gemelli dell efficacia dell acido orotico quale fattore di
        crescita. Acta Vitaminol., 16, 193–198 (1962)

S21   Shafritz, D. A. and Senior, J. R. Synthesis of pyrimidine
        nucleotide precursors in human and rat small intestinal
        mucosa. Biochim. Biophys. Acta, 141, 332–341 (1967)

S22   Shevtsov, V. V., Glebov, R. N., Mezentsev, A. N. and
        Pogodaev, K. I. Effects of repetitive electroconvulsions on
        incorporation of lysine-[^{3}H] and orotic-[^{14}C] acid into sub-
        cellular fractions of rat brain cortex in long-term experi-
        ments. Vopr. Med. Khim., 18, 467–471 (1972) (Russ.)

S23   Shushevich, S. I., Khalmuradov, A. G. and Shestopalova,
        V. M. Vliianie orotovoi kisloty na soderzhanie piridinovykh
        kofermentov v tkani pecheni krys. Vopr. Med. Khim., 13,
        136–139 (1967)

S24   Sickinger, K., Kattermann, R. and Hannemann, H. Zunahme von Lebergewicht und Leberglykogen unter Infusion von Cholinorotat und Adenosin. Acta Hepato Splenol., 14, 88–99 (1967)

S25   Sidransky, H., Verney, E. and Wagle, D. S. Effect of dietary orotic acid on liver glycogen. Proc. Soc. Exp. Biol. Med., 120 (1965)

S26   Sidransky, H. and Verney, E. Chronic fatty liver without cirrhosis induced in the rat by dietary orotic acid. Am. J. Pathol., 46, 1007–1013 (1965)

S27   Sidransky, H. and Verney, E. Influence of orotic acid on liver tumorigenesis in rats ingesting ethionine, N-2-fluorenylacetamide and 3'-methyl-dimethylaminoazobenzene. J. Natl. Cancer Inst., 44, 1201–1215 (1970)

S28   Simmonds, H. A., Potter, C. F., Sahota, A., Cameron, J. S., Webster, D. R. and Becroft, D. M. O. Absence of orotic aciduria in adenosine deaminase deficiency and purine nucleoside phosphorylase deficiency. Clin. Exp. Immunol., 34, 42–45 (1978)

S29   Simon, J. B., Scheig, R. and Klatskin, G. Protection by orotic acid against the renal necrosis and fatty liver of choline deficiency. Proc. Soc. Exp. Biol. Med., 129, 874–877 (1968)

S30   Simon, J. B., Scheig, R. and Klatskin, G. Hepatic ATP and triglyceride levels in choline-deficient rats with and without dietary orotic acid supplementation. J. Nutr., 98, 188–192 (1969)

S31   Simonson, E. and Berman, R. New approach in treatment of cardiac decompensation in USSR. Am. Heart J., 86, 117–123 (1973)

S32   Smith, L. H. Jr., Huguley, Ch., M. Jr. and Brain, J. A. Hereditary orotic aciduria. In The Metabolic Basis of Inherited Disease. 3rd edn., pp. 1003–1029 (1972)

S33   Smith, L. H. and Gilmour, L. Determination of urinary carbamylaspartate and dihydroorotate in normal subjects and in patients with hereditary orotic aciduria. J. Lab. Clin. Med., 86, 1047–1051 (1975)

S34   Smith, P. C., Knott, Ch. E. and Trembly, G. C. Detection of the feedback control of pyrimidine biosynthesis in slices of several rat tissues. Biochem. Biophys. Res. Commun., 55, 1141–1146 (1973)

S35   Sociéte de Recherche de Biologie Thérapeutique. Purine Orotate Hepatic Protectors and Tissue Regenerators. Fr. M4094 (Cl. A61k, CO7d), May 23, 1966 Appl. Dec. 1, 1964, 2 pp.

S36   Solomin, V. G. and Ivanov, V. Ya. Effect of orotic acid and an extract of Biberstein carline thistle on lactate dehydrogenase and alkaline phosphatase activities under an increased physical load. Farmakol. Reparation. Regeneratsu, 3, 63–67 (1977). From Ref. Zh. Biol. Khim. (1977) (Russ.) Abstr. No. 23Ch 368

S37   Soutter, G. B., Yu, J. S., Lovric, A. and Stapleton, T. Hereditary orotic aciduria. Aust. Paediatr. J., 6, 47 (1970)

S38   Spiegel, A. J. and Noseworthy, M. M. Use of nonaqueous solvents in parenteral products. J. Pharm. Sci., 52, 917–927 (1963)

S39   Sung, M. T., Dixon, G. H. and Smithies, O. Phosphorylation and synthesis of histones in regenerating rat liver. J. Biol. Chem., 246, 1358–1364 (1971)

S40   Sunshine, Ph., Lindenbaum, J. E., Levy, H. L. and Freeman, J. M. Hyperammonemia due to a defect in hepatic ornithine transcarbamylase. Pediatrics, 50, 100–111 (1972)

S41   Svetlavivienc, L. Effect of orotic acid on blood serum aminotransferase activity in experimental fascioliasis of sheep previously freed from helminths. Presented at the 7th Probl. Parazitol. Tr. Nauch. Konf. Parazitol. Ukr. SSR, 2, 235–236 (1972) (Russ.)

S42   Sweeney, M. J. and Hoffman, D. H. Dihydroorotate dehydrogenase in liver and Morris hepatomas. Cancer Res., 33, 394–396 (1973)

S43   Szam, I., Fischer, J., Gulyas, A., Hagedüs-Wein, I., Hollo, J., Karpati, P., Kisfaludy, S., Szentner, I., Szilard, T. and Vass, A. Tierexperimentelle und klinische Beiträge zur Pathophysiologie und Therapie des Ammoniakstoffwechsels. Presented at the 2te Internationale Ammoniakkonferenz, May (1974) Strasbourg

S44   Szelenyi, I., Sos, J., Rigo, J. and Surtya, M. Effect of magnesium orotate and orotic acid on experimental hypertension and cardiopathogenic changes in heart muscle. Dtsch. Med. J., 21 and 22, 1405–1406, 1409–1410 and 1412 (1970) (Germ.)

S45   Szelenyi, I. Wirkung von Magnesium-Orotat und Orotsäure auf die Enzymaktivität der Leber. Experimentelle Untersuchungen. Münch. Med. Wochensch. 112, 1516–1519 (1970)

S46   Szelenyi, I., Nemesanszky, E., Nagy, Z., Li Bok Nam, Romics, I. and Rigo, J. Experimentelle Leberschäden und ihre Beeinflussung durch anorganische und organische Magnesium-Salze. Arzneim. Forsch., 21, 772–777 (1971)

S47   Szelenyi, I., Pucsok, J., Nemesanszky, E. and Sos, J. Pathophysiologische Untersuchungen zum Lipoidmetabolismus der Leber unter der Wirkung von Orotsäure und Magnesium-Orotat. Arzneim. Forsch., 21, 777–779 (1971)

S48   Szelenyi, I., Nemesanszky, E., Laszlo, G. and Desi, J. Wirkung von Magnesium-Orotat-Glycinat auf die experimentelle Ammoniak-Intoxikation. Arzneim. Forsch., 21, 787–788 (1971)

S49   Szelenyi, I., Farkas, I., Desi, I. and Nemesanszky, E. Effect of magnesium orotate glycinate on the brain electric activity after experimental ammonia poisoning. Arzneim. Forsch., 21, 789–791 (1971) (Germ.)

S50   Szirmai, E. and Klosa, J. Der Einfluss wasserlöslicher Orotsäure den Lernprozess von Ratten. Arzneim. Forsch., 26, 1685–1686 (1976)

Sch

S51   Scharnbeck, H., Schaffner, F., Keppler, D. and Decker, D. Ultrastructural studies on the effect of choline orotate on galactosamine induced hepatic injury in rats. Exp. Mol. Pathol., 16, 33–46 (1972)

S52   Schmid, W. and Sekeris, C. E. Kontrolle der nucleolaren RNA-Synthese durch DNA-ähnliche RNA. Hoppe-Seyler's Z. Physiol. Chem., 353, 1564 (1972)

S53   Schmidt, B. J., Ramos, A. O., Caldeira, J. A. F. and Monteiro, D. C. M. Orotic acid and experimental galactosemia. J. Pediatr., 68, 138–139 (1966)

S54   Schrader, K. E., Beneke, G., Rommel, K. and Mähr, G. Einfluss der Orotsäure auf die experimentelle Galaktose Katarakt mit histochemischen Untersuchungsergebnissen: Albrecht von Graefes Arch. Klin. Exp. Ophthalmol. 168, 358–364 (1965)

S55   Schulzeck, S., Schmidt, S., Pohle, W. and Popov, N. Separation and detection of orotic acid in plasma, urine, and tissues. Z. Med. Labortech., 12, 193–198 (1971) (Germ.)

S56   Schwarze, R., Kintzel, H. W. and Hinkel, G. K. The influence of orotic acid on the serum bilirubin level of mature newborn. Acta Paediatr. Scand., 60, 705–708 (1971)

S57   Schwietzer, C. H. Die Bedeutung von Purinkörpern für die Lebertherapie. Verh. Dtsch. Ges. Inn. Med., 59, 311–312 (1953)

S58   Schwietzer, C. H., Physiologische Eigenschaften der Orotsäure. Biochem. Z., 328, 291–300 (1956)

St

S59   Stajner, A., Suva, J. and Musil, F. The determination of orotic acid in the blood serum by means of the spectrophotometric method. Experientia, 24, 116–117 (1968)

S60   Standerfer, S. B. and Handler, Ph. Fatty liver induced by orotic acid feeding. Proc. Soc. Exp. Biol. Med., 90, 270–271 (1955)

S61   Statter, M., Russel, A., Abzug-Horowitz, S. and Pinson, A. Abnormal orotic acid metabolism associated with acute hyperammonaemia in the rat. Biochem. Med., 9, 1–18 (1974)

S62   Stirpe, F. and Fiume, L. Studies on the pathogenesis of liver necrosis by α-amanitin. Effect of α-amanitin on ribonucleic acid synthesis and on ribonucleic acid polymerase in mouse liver nuclei. Biochem. J., 105, 779–782 (1967)

S63   Stomonyakova, S., Novachev., D. and Todorova, K. Serum enzyme activities in newborn infants treated with orotic acid. Pediatriya (Sofia), 15, 44–49 (1976) (Bulg.)

S64   Stone, J. E. and Hough, A. J. Simple systems for the investigation of the effects of drugs upon uridine nucleotide metabolism. Behav. Neuropsychiatry, 3, 8–14 and 24 (1972)

S65   Strzalka, K. Effect of light on the incorporation of carbon-14-labelled orotic acid by wheat seedlings. Bull. Acad. Pol. Sci., Ser. Sci. Biol., 23, 243–247 (1975)

T

T1   Takahashi, T. and Fujisawa, K. The effect of various nucleotides on experimental fatty liver and hepatic damage. Jikeikai Med. J., 13, 143–152 (1966)

T2   Tanaka, T., Takagi, M. and Ogata, K. Metabolism of RNA of free and membrane-bound polysomes from rat liver. Biochim. Biophys. Acta, 224, 507–517 (1970)

T3   Tax, W. J. M., Veerkamp, J. H. and Schretlen, E. D. A. M. The urinary excretion of orotic acid and orotidine, measured by an isotope dilution assay. Clin. Chim. Acta, 90, 209 (1978)

T4   Tay, W. J. M., Veerkamp, J. H., Trijbels, F. J. M. and Schretlen, E. D. A. M. Mechanism of allopurinol-mediated inhibition and stabilization of human orotate phosphoribosyltransferase and orotidine phosphate decarboxylase. Biochem. Pharmacol., 25, 2025–2032 (1976)

T5   Tereschenko, O. Ya. Analysis of labeled orotic acid metabolites excretion as a means of studying the metabolism of nuclear compounds. Biokhimiya, 32, 462–470 (1967) (Russ.)

T6   Tezuka, M. and Tamemasa, O. Incorporation characteristics of uracil, uridine and orotic acid into ribonucleic acid of neoplastic cells. Gann, 68, 287–292 (1977)

T7   Thomas, H. M. Inhibition of ethanol toxicity by lysine orotate (ORL). FEBS Lett., 7, 291–292 (1970)

T8   Thrower, S., Ord, M. G. and Stocken, L. A. Effects of phenoxybenzamine on early stages of liver regeneration in partially hepatectomized rats. Biochem. Pharmacol., 22, 95–100 (1973)

T9   Tomarelli, R. M., Bauman, L. M. and Weaber, J. R. Protective effect of milk against orotic acid fatty liver. Presented at the Second Joint Meeting of the American Institute of Nutrition, the American Society for Clinical Nutrition, and the Nutrition Society of Canada. August 8–11 (1976) Michigan State University

T10   Torrielli, M. V. and Ugazio, G. Effect of DPPD on the orotic acid-induced fatty liver in the rat. Life Sci., II, 1–7 (1970)

T11   Torrielli, M. V., Dianzani, M. U. and Ugazio, G. Behaviour of lipoperoxidation in rat liver during orotic acid treatment. Life Sci., II, 99–111 (1971)

T12   Trager, W. Malaria parasites (*Plasmodium lophurae*) developing extracellularly – *in vitro* incorporation of labeled precursors. J. Protozool., 18, 392–399 (1971)

T13   Trapmann, H. and Devani, M. Orotsäure—ein biogener Wirkstoff. Dtsch. Apoth. Z., 105, 313–316 (1965)

T14   Traut, T. W. Inhibitors of orotate phosphoribosyltransferase and orotidine-5'-phosphate decarboxylase from mouse Ehrlich ascites cells: a procedure for analyzing the inhibition of a multi-enzyme complex. Biochem. Pharmacol., 26, 2291–2296 (1977)

T15   Tremblay, G. C., Crandall, D. E., Knott, Ch. E. and Alfant, M. Orotic acid biosynthesis in rat liver: studies on the source of carbamoylphosphate. Arch. Biochem. Biophys., 178, 264–277 (1977)

T16   Tsang, D. and Johnstone, R. M. Steroidogenesis and RNA synthesis in rat adrenal gland *in vitro*. Endocrinology, 93, 119–126 (1973)

T17 Tseng, J. K. and Gurpide, E. Compartmentalization of uridine and uridine-5'-monophosphate in rat liver slices. J. Biol. Chem., 248, 5634–5640 (1973)

T18 Tubergen, D. K., Krooth, R. S. and Heyn, R. M. Hereditary orotic aciduria with normal growth and development. Am. J. Dis. Child., 118, 864–870 (1969)

U

U1 Uchida, M., Ohara, A. and Yamazaki, M. The effect of orotic acid on the synthesis of glucuronides. Takamine Kenyusho Nempo, 11, 137–141 (1959) (Japan.)

U2 Unarova, S. A. Antiinflammatory action of potassium orotate and its mechanism. Dokl. Akad. Nauk Tadzh. SSR, 18, 64–67 (1975) (Russ.)

V

V1 Vacha, J. and Seifert, J. Turnover of cytidine and uridine components of acid-soluble pool and RNA of cytoplasmic ribosomes after repeated phenobarbital administration. Biochem. Pharmacol., 24, 401–405 (1975)

V2 Vaishwanar, I. and Jiddewar, G. G. Orotic acid induced fatty liver and influence of papain. Indian J. Biochem., 7, 214 (1970)

V3 Valli, E. A., Sarma, D. S. R. and Sarma, P. S. Species specificity in orotic acid induced fatty liver. Indian J. Biochem., 5, 120–122 (1968)

V4 Varshavskii, B. Ya., Verlinskii, S. G. and Biryulya, V. A. Effect of potassium orotate on the transport of organic substances in the kidneys. Byull. Eksp. Biol. Med., 77, 58–60 (1974) (Russ.)

V5   Vasseur, J. Incorporation of [^{14}C] orotic acid and [^{14}C] uracil into ribonucleotides of chicory leaf fragments grown *in vitro*. C. R. Acad. Sci. Ser. D., 275, 2865–2868 (1972) (Fr.)

V6   Velyanov, D., Raducheva, T., Maneva, L. and Golovinski, E. Influence of the hydrazides of precursors of the pyrimidine mononucleotides on the respiration of *Escherichia coli*. Dokl. Bolg. Akad. Nauk., 30, 285–287 (1977)

V7   Verga, A. L'acido orotico come fattore di crescita nell'immaturo. Minerva Pediatr., 12, 1006–1007 (1960)

V8   Vest, M. Phototherapie senkt Serumbilirubin. Reifung der Bilirubinkonjugation und Gallenfarbstoff Exkretion nicht gefördert. Med. Tribune (1972)

V9   Villanyi, P., Votin, J. and Rahlfs, V. Arteriosclerosis, myocardial infarct and blood lipids; their therapeutic modification by magnesium orotate. Wien. Med. Wochenschr., 120, 76–83 (1970) (Germ.)

V10 Villari, V. and Mazzacca, G. Il sale potassico dell'acido orotico nell'infezione sperimentale da virus MHV-3 (Mouse Hepatitis Virus). Acta Vitaminol., 12, 69–72 (1958)

V11 Villela, G. G. and Jansen, S. Effect of cerebral extracts on the degradation of orotates. Rev. Bras. Biol., 35, 509–513 (Port.)

V12 Vitol, M. I. A., Shaposhinkov, V. N. K. and Shvachkin, I. U. P. New route of catabolism of orotic acid in microorganisms. Dokl. Akad. Nauk. SSSR, 174, 1202–1204 (1967) (Russ.)

V13 Viviani, R., Marchetti, M., Rabbi, A. and Moruzzi, G. Relationship between orotic acid and animal protein factors of casein. Nature (London), 176, 464 (1955)

V14 Viviani, R., Sechi, A. M. and Moruzzi, G. Effect of orotic acid in lysine-deficient rats. Int. Z. Vitaminforsch., 30, 95–97 (1969)

V15 Vogt, H. Orotsäure im Geflügelfutter. Arch. Geflügelkd., 3, 96–102 (1976)

V16 Volokhov, A. A. and Serebryakova, L. I. Acquisition and retention of a conditioned avoidance reflex in rats developing prenatally under the effect of orotic acid. In Omani, T. N. (ed.) Mekh. Devat. Golown. Mozga, pp. 120–125 (1975) (Tiflis, USSR)

W

W1   Wallnöfer, H. Die Behandlung der Hepatosen. Muench. Med. Wochenschr., 114, 186–190 (1972)

W2   Walther, H., Meyer, F. P. and Koehler, E. Pharmacokinetics of orotic acid in adults and children. Zentralbl. Pharm. Pharmakother. Laboratoriumsdiagn, 115, 615–619 (1976)

W3   Waxin, B. S. Etude pharmacologique et clinique d'une médication associant acide orotique et sorbitol dans les affections hépato-biliaires. Thesis, Faculté de Médécine de Paris (1969)

W4   Weissman, S. M., Eisen, A. Z., Fallon, H., Lewis, M. and Karon, M. The metabolism of ring-labeled orotic acid in man. J. Clin. Invest., 41, 1546–1552 (1962)

W5   Wenzel, E. Der therapeutische Einfluss von Kavain und Magnesium-Orotat auf traumatisch- und gefässbedingte Hirnschäden. Wien. Med. Wochenschr., 121, 226–236 (1971)

W6   White, H. H. and Ross, L. Detection of orotic acid by thin-layer chromatography. Tech. Bull. Regist. Med. Technol., 39, 275–277 (1969)

W7   Wildhirt, E. Die Behandlung der akuten Virushepatitis mit orotsaurem Cholin. Ther. Umsch. 19, 387–390 (1962)

W8   Wildhirt, E. and Selmair, H. Neue Erfahrungen bei der Behandlung der akuten Virus-Hepatitis—die Wirkung von Cholinorotat. Muench. Med. Wochenschr., 109, 887–891 (1967)

W9   Wildhirt, E. Hepatitis-Therapie ohne Nebenwirkungen. Prax. Kurier, 12, (1967)

W10   Wildhirt, E., Klinik und Therapie der chronischen Hepatitis. Die Heilkunst, Z. Prakt. Med. 83, 1–16 (1970)

W11 Wildhirt, E. Die Bedeutung der Orotsäure in der Lebertherapie. Informierte Arzt, 4, 18–21 (1976)

W12 Wildhirt, E. Trends in der Diagnostik von Leberkrankheiten. Prax. Kurier, 2 (Suppl.), 12 (1976)

W13 Wilkinson, D. S., Čihak, A. and Pitot, H. C. Inhibition of ribosomal ribonucleic acid maturation in rat liver by 5-fluoroorotic acid resulting in the selective labeling of cytoplasmic messenger ribonucleic acid. J. Biol. Chem., 246, 6418–6427 (1971)

W14 Williams, J. F., Donohoe, J., Lykke, A. and Kolos, G. Studies using orotic acid for improving the controlled development of myocardial hypertrophy. Aust. N.Z. J. Med., 6, 60–71 (1976) 1 (1976)

W15 Windmueller, H. G. An orotic acid-induced, adenine-reversed inhibition of hepatic lipoprotein secretion in the rat. J. Biol. Chem., 239, 530–537 (1964)

W16 Windmueller, H. G. and Spaeth, A. E. Stimulation of hepatic purine biosynthesis by orotic acid. J. Biol. Chem., 240, 4398–4405 (1965)

W17 Windmueller, H. G., McDaniel, E. G. and Spaeth, A. Orotic acid-induced fatty liver. Metabolic studies in conventional and germ-free rats. Arch. Biochem. Biophys., 109, 13–19 (1965)

W18 Windmueller, H. G. and Spaeth, A. E. Perfusion *in situ* with tritum oxide to measure hepatic lipogenesis and lipid secretion. J. Biol. Chem., 241, 2891–2899 (1966)

W19 Windmueller, H. G. and Spaeth, A. E. *De novo* synthesis of fatty acid in perfused rat liver as a determinant of plasma lipoprotein production. Arch. Biochem. Biophys., 122, 362–369 (1967)

W20 Windmueller, H. G. and Levy, R. I. Total inhibition of hepatic β-lipoprotein production in the rat by orotic acid. J. Biol. Chem., 242, 2246–2254 (1967)

W21 Windmueller, H. G., Levy, R. I. and Spaeth, A. E. Selective inhibition of hepatic, but not intestinal β-

lipoprotein production and triglyceride transport in rats given orotic acid. Adv. Exp. Med. Biol., 4, 365–375 (1969)

W22   Windmueller, H. G. and von Euler, L. H. Prevention of orotic acid-induced fatty liver with allopurinol. Proc. Soc. Exp. Biol. Med., 136, 98–101 (1971)

W23   Witschi, H.-P. A comparative study *in vivo* RNA and protein synthesis in rat liver and lung. Cancer Res., 32, 1686–1694 (1972)

W24   Witschi, H.-P. Qualitative and quantitative aspects of the biosynthesis of ribonucleic acid and of protein in the liver and the lung of the Syrian golden hamster. Biochem. J., 136, 781–788 (1973)

W25   Witting, L. A. Fatty liver induction inverse relationship between hepatic neutral lipid accumulation and dietary polyunsaturated fatty acids in orotic acid-fed rats. J. Lipid Res., 13, 27–31 (1972)

W26   Witting, L. A. Fatty liver induction. Effect of ethionine on polyunsaturated fatty acid synthesis. Biochim. Biophys. Acta, 296, 271–286 (1973)

W27   Wood, M. H., Sebel, E. and O'Sullivan, W. J. Allopurinol and thiazides. Lancet, 1, 751 (1972)

W28   Wood, M. H. and O'Sullivan, W. J. The orotic aciduria of pregnancy. Am. J. Obstet. Gynecol., 116, 57–61 (1973)

W29   Worthy, Th. E., Grobner, W. and Kelley, W. N. Hereditary orotic aciduria. Evidence for a structural gene mutation. Proc. Natl. Acad. Sci. USA, 71, 3031–3035 (1974)

Y

Y1   Yamada, T., Yamaguchi, M., Kuroiwa, S. and Ito, M. The effect of AICA orotate in the treatment of liver diseases. Asian Med. J., 8, 357–372 (1965)

Y2   Yatvin, M. B. and Abdel - Halim, M. N. Liver RNA

metabolism in adrenalectomized and intact whole-body irradiated and 5-fluoroorotic acid treated rats. Int. J. Radiat. Oncol. Biol. Phys., 1, 945–950 (1976)

Y3   Yngner, T., Lewan, L. and Petersen, I. Factors influencing the serum activity in mice after intravenous and intraperitoneal injection of [^{14}C] orotic acid. Experientia, 31, 387–388 (1975)

Y4   Yoneda, S., Carvalho, R. P. de S. and Castellani, B. R. Synthesis of pyrimidine base by intracellular forms of *Toxoplasma gondii* in cell culture. Rev. Inst. Med. Trop. Sao Paulo, 16, 328–331 (1974)

Y5   Yousufzai, S. Y. K.   and   Siddiqi,   M.   3-Hydroxy-3-methylglutaric acid and orotic acid induced fatty liver in rats. Lipids, 12, 689–690 (1977)

Y6   Yu, Fu-Li and Feigelson, Ph. Effects of cortisone on orotic acid transport and RNA synthesis in rat liver. Arch. Biochem. Biophys., 141, 662–667 (1970)

Z

Z1   Zabrodin, O. N. Pharmacological analysis of the participation of endogenous norepinephrine in the retrograde development of neurogenic gastric dystrophy. Farmakol. Toksikol. 35, 606–610 (1972) (Russ.)

Z2   Zaki, F. G. Fatty cirrhosis in the rat. XII. The cirrhotic nodules. Arch. Pathol., 81, 536–543 (1966)

Z3   Zakim, D. The effect of orotic acid feeding on hepatic phospholipid metabolism. Fed. Proc., 26, 412 (1967)

Z4   Zarina, L., Blugere, N. and Snikeris, D. Effect of salts of dihydroorotic acid on the structure and function of white rat liver in chronic intoxication with tetrachloromethane. Latv. PSR Zinat. Akad. Vestis, 1, 71–74 (1975) (Russ.)

Z5   Zharov, E. I., Markovskaya, G. I. and Iurasov, V. S. Effect of the cofactors of synthesis and precursors of nucleic acids on the state of the myocardium in myocardial infarct according to electrocardiographic data. Kardiologiia, 8, 59–64 (1968) (Russ.)

Z6   Zharov, E. I. Use of cofactors of the synthesis and precursors of nucleic acids in myocardial infarct patients. Kardiologiia, 11, 15–25 (1971) (Russ.)

Z7   Zhivkov, V. and Geshanova, E. [14C]-Precursors incorporation into adenine and uridine nucleotides of the liver of some vertebrates. Comp. Biochem. Physiol., 50, 165–167 (1975)

Z8   Zhivkov, V. The measurement of the rate of synthesis of uridine diphosphate sugars in animal tissues by [14C] orotate incorporation. Int. J. Biochem. 9, 89–92 (1978) .

Z9   Zhukova, S. V., Blagodatskaya, V. M. and Odintsova, E. N. The effects of some vitamins on the synthesis of nucleic acids and other phosphorus compounds in yeast cells in the lag phase. Dokl. Akad. Nauk. SSSR, 173, 1438–1440 (1967) (Russ.)

Z10   Zimmer, V. Die Wirkung von Amino-imidazol-karboxamid-orotat bei Lebererkrankungen. Aerztl. Prax., 23, 3411–3412 (1971)

Z11   Zöllner, N. and Gröbner, W. Influence of oral ribonucleic acid on oroticaciduria due to allopurinol administration. Z. Gesamte. Exp. Med., 156, 317–319 (1971)

Z12   Zöllner, N., Janssen, A. and Gröbner, W. Partielle Aufhebung der Allopurinolinduzierten Orotacidurie durch Ribonucleotide. Presented at the 81st Tag. Dtsch. Ges. Inn. Med. (Wiesbaden), April 6–10 (1975).

Z13   Zöllner, N. and Gröbner, W. Der Einfluss verschiedener Purin- und Pyrimidinnukleoside auf die Pyrimidinsythese des Menschen. Presented at the 84th Tag. Dtsch. Ges. Inn. Med. (Wiesbaden), April 2–6 (1978)

Z14   Zoltan, T. Ö and Baldizsar, M. Beeinflussung zerebraler Ernährungsstörungen durch Kavain und Magnesium-Orotat. Acta Gerontol., 9, 525–530 (1971)

Z15   Zoltan, T. Ö. and Baldizsar, M. Die protektive Wirkung von Kavain und Magnesiumorotat bei neurotoxischer Belastung des Zentralnervensystems durch Strychnin. Acta. Gerontol., 2, 243–245 (1972)

INDEX

OROTIC ACID

Uridine   A8, B11, G1, H18, M23,
   R5, T6, T17

Vitamin A   B1, D2
Vitamin B$_{12}$ C2, C3, C4, C5, D9,
   D10, H15, H16, K52, M7, M9,

M12, M47, P8, P9
Vitamin E   B44, C19

Xanthine A1

Zinc N14